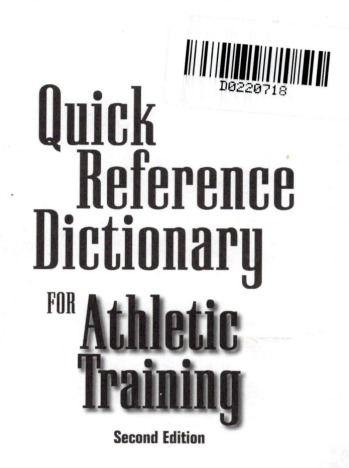

Quick Reference Dictionary
FOR Athletic Training

Second Edition

Quick Reference Dictionary

FOR Athletic Training

Second Edition

Julie N. Bernier, EdD, ATC
Plymouth State University
Plymouth, NH

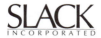

SLACK
INCORPORATED

An innovative information, education, and management company
6900 Grove Road • Thorofare, NJ 08086

ISBN-10: 1-55642-666-6
ISBN-13: 978-1-55642-666-7

The procedures and practices described in this book should be implemented in a manner consistent with the professional standards set for the circumstances that apply in each specific situation. Every effort has been made to confirm the accuracy of the information presented and to correctly relate generally accepted practices. The author, editor, and publisher cannot accept responsibility for errors or exclusions or for the outcome of the application of the material presented herein. There is no expressed or implied warranty of this book or information imparted by it.

The work SLACK publishes is peer reviewed. Prior to publication, recognized leaders in the field, educators, and clinicians provide important feedback on the concepts and content that we publish. We welcome feedback on this work.

Printed in the United States of America.

Library of Congress Cataloging-in-Publication Data

Bernier, Julie N., 1964-
  Quick reference dictionary for athletic training / Julie N. Bernier.-- 2nd ed.
    p. ; cm.
  Includes bibliographical references.
  ISBN-13: 978-1-55642-666-7 (alk. paper)
  ISBN-10: 1-55642-666-6 (alk. paper)
  1. Physical education and training--Dictionaries.
    [DNLM: 1. Physical Education and Training--Dictionary--English. 2. Athletic Injuries--Dictionary--English. 3. Musculoskeletal Physiology--Dictionary--English.] I. Title.

RC1206.B475 2005
617.1'027'03--dc22
                                                2004028843

Published by: SLACK Incorporated
                       6900 Grove Road
                       Thorofare, NJ 08086 USA
                       Telephone: 856-848-1000
                       Fax: 856-853-5991
                       www.slackbooks.com

Contact SLACK Incorporated for more information about other books in this field or about the availability of our books from distributors outside the United States.

For permission to reprint material in another publication, contact SLACK Incorporated. Authorization to photocopy items for internal, personal, or academic use is granted by SLACK Incorporated provided that the appropriate fee is paid directly to Copyright Clearance Center. Prior to photocopying items, please contact the Copyright Clearance Center at 222 Rosewood Drive, Danvers, MA 01923 USA; phone: 978-750-8400; website: www.copyright.com; email: info@copyright.com.

For further information on CCC, check CCC Online at the following address: http://www.copyright.com.

Last digit is print number: 10   9   8   7   6   5   4   3   2   1

DEDICATION

This book is dedicated to my mentor and very good friend David H. Perrin.

CONTENTS

ACKNOWLEDGMENTS

I wish to extend my sincere gratitude to the people at SLACK Incorporated, especially Amy McShane, Debra Toulson, Carrie Kotlar, Michelle Gatt, and Megan Charlton. I want to thank Marge Albohm, who suggested I take on this project. My sincere thanks to Karen and Laela Jacobs and Jennifer Bottomley for providing the inspiration with the *Quick Reference Dictionary for Occupational Therapy* and *Quick Reference Dictionary for Physical Therapy*. I must thank my colleagues for putting up with me when I take on these projects and my students for inspiring me every day and reminding me why I came into this profession. Lastly, I would like to thank the four most influential mentors in my life: David H. Perrin, PhD, ATC, Sherry Bovinet, PhD, ATC, Charlie Beach, PhD, and Dorothy Diehl, PhD.

About the Editor

Julie N. Bernier, EdD, ATC is the Associate Vice President for Academic Affairs at Plymouth State University. She previously served as Department Chair of Health and Human Performance and Director of graduate and undergraduate Athletic Training at Plymouth State University in Plymouth, NH, where she has been since 1988. Julie received her bachelor of science and master of education degrees from Keene State College in New Hampshire and her doctorate from the University of Virginia. She serves on the editorial board of the Journal of Athletic Training and has served on numerous NATA and NATA-REF committees. In her other life she is a potter and also enjoys building furniture.

INTRODUCTION

This book is intended to serve as a reference tool for clinicians and students of athletic training. It provides quick reference to over 2100 terms related to the field of athletic training. Additionally, it contains 20 appendices that I hope you will find useful.

Appendices 1 to 3 were written to aid the practitioner or student in writing progress notes and includes a table of medical root terminology, acronyms and abbreviations, and symbols commonly used by practitioners. Appendices 4 through 11 serve as an anatomical reference for the student. Appendix 4 includes anatomical terms. Appendix 5 provides figures of the superficial and deep muscles of the body followed by a table that includes origin, insertion, action, and nerve innervations. Appendix 6 is new to this edition and covers manual muscle testing, which includes patient positioning, examiner stabilization, and patient action. Appendix 7 provides a table of normal joint ranges of motion. Appendix 8 provides a review of cranial nerves. Appendix 9 includes information on grading systems for assessment of concussion, while Appendices 10 through 13 cover nerve root assessment and peripheral nerve innervations. Appendices 14 and 15 provide assessment scales for grades of pain and normal and abnormal end feels. Appendix 16 has bee added in this edition and provides reference to loose and tight packed positions for joint mobilization. The most comprehensive section, Appendix 17, provides information for more than 85 orthopedic special tests. Appendix 18 provides an overview of commonly used prescription medications. Appendix 19 provides quick access to pertinent NATA membership standard and Code of Ethics. Finally, Appendix 20 provides reference to conversion of weights and measures.

A

A β fiber (A beta): An afferent nerve fiber that is stimulated by touch, pressure, tension, movement, and vibration.

A δ fiber (A delta): An afferent neuron responsible for carrying temperature and noxious stimuli; responsible for "fast pain."

abdomen, acute: Acute onset of abdominal pain due to any number of causes including appendicitis, cholecystitis, perforated ulcer, and ruptured spleen.

abdominal aneurysm: An aneurysm within the abdomen. *See* aneurysm.

abdominal cavity: The cavity formed between the abdominal wall and the spine that houses a number of organs including the stomach, colon, small intestine, liver, gallbladder, pancreas, spleen, kidneys, bladder, and rectum.

abdominal guarding: Involuntary contraction of the abdominal muscles to protect organs in response to injury or illness to one or more organs.

abdominal quadrants: Four divisions of the abdomen determined by drawing imaginary vertical and horizontal lines through the umbilicus. The upper left quadrant contains the stomach, spleen, and pancreas; upper right contains the liver and gallbladder; lower right contains the appendix; and lower left contains the colon.

abducens nerve: Cranial nerve VI; innervates the lateral rectus femoris muscle of the eye, responsible for lateral eye movement. *See* Appendix 8.

abduct: To move away from the midline in the frontal plane.

abduction (ABD): Movement of a body part (usually the limbs) away from the midline of the body.

abductor muscle: A muscle whose primary responsibility is to abduct the limb.

abrasion: Minor wound in skin surface, caused by rubbing or scraping.

abscess: Collection of pus.

absolute refractory period: The period following depolarization in which another action potential cannot occur.

absorption: The taking in of liquids, gases, or light.

acceleration: The change in velocity per unit of time (meters per second per second-m/s^2). For example, 1 m/s^2 means that velocity is increased by 1 m/s every second. *See also* gravity.

accessory motion: Also called secondary motion. The small motions of sliding, spinning, and rolling that are necessary in order to have physiological (primary) motion.

accessory movers: Muscles that assist the prime movers in performing a function.

accessory nerve: Cranial nerve XI responsible for the innervation of the sternocleidomastoid and the trapezius muscles. *See* Appendix 8.

acclimatization: To adapt to a new temperature, climate, environment, or situation; the act of adapting to altitude, usually taking 1 to 3 days for each change in altitude.

accommodating resistance: As in the resistance given by an isokinetic dynamometer. The resistance supplied by the dynamometer is equal to the resistance put in by the patient.

accommodation: Adaptation; adjustment; the act of adjusting to a stimulus.

ACE inhibitor: A drug that inhibits the formation of angiotensin II; used to treat high blood pressure.

acetabulum: The "cup-shaped" socket of the hip joint that articulates with the head of the femur.

acetaminophen: A pain-relieving drug commonly known as Tylenol (McNeil Consumer & Specialty Pharmaceuticals, Ft. Washington, Pa).

acetylsalicylic acid: Aspirin; a nonsteroidal anti-inflammatory used for the relief of pain and fever.

achalasia: A disease of the esophagus in which the ability to swallow is impaired.

Achilles' tendon: The distal insertion of the gastrocnemius and soleus muscles into the plantar surface of the calcaneus; Syn: calcaneal tendon.

ACI: *See* approved clinical instructor.

acid reflux: *See* gastroesophageal reflux.

acid-base balance: Refers to the control of pH in which the body's fluids are neither acidic nor alkaline.

acidosis: An abnormal condition in which the pH is too low (ie, becomes acidic); caused by diabetes, kidney disease, or lung disease; leads to ketoacidosis in the diabetic individual.

AC joint (acromioclavicular joint): The articulation between the acromion process (the distal end of the spine of the scapula) and the lateral end of the clavicle. The acromioclavicular ligament forms the capsular ligament while the trapezoid and conoid ligaments (coracoclavicular ligaments) strengthen this articulation.

acne vulgaris: A skin condition that most commonly affects adolescents; characterized by pus-filled pimples on the skin caused by overactivity of the oil glands.

acoustical spectrum: A means of displaying the range of frequencies and wavelengths of sound waves. Ultrasound is a form of radiation classified in the acoustical spectrum.

acquired: A condition not contracted at birth but one that later develops.

acquired immunodeficiency syndrome (AIDS): Disease of the immune system caused by the human immunodeficiency virus (HIV).

acromegaly: A disease in which there is continued production of growth hormone by the pituitary gland after the end of adolescence.

acromion: The distal end of the spine of the scapula that forms the top of the shoulder.

acromion process: The superior lateral process of the spine of the scapula that articulates with the clavicle and forms the "top" of the shoulder.

acromioplasty: The surgical removal of the inferior distal end of the acromion process of the scapula; a procedure used to relieve soft tissue impingement in the subacromial space.

AC shear test: AC joint compression test. Test to examine the integrity of the AC joint. *See* Special Tests—Shoulder (Appendix 17).

action potential: The change in voltage across the membrane of nerve or muscle.

active assistive range of motion (AAROM): Movement at a joint achieved by muscular contraction of the agonist muscles with assistance.

active electrode: In electrical stimulation, in which a monopolar pad placement is used (two pads of unequal size), it is the smaller of the two pads placed over the injured site, trigger point, motor point, or nerve.

active range of motion (AROM): Movement at a joint achieved by muscular contraction of the agonist muscles.

activities of daily living (ADLs): The skills required for independence in everyday living including activities such as mobility and self-care.

acuity test, visual: A test to measure the clarity of vision; *See also* Snellen's chart.

acupressure: Pressure applied to trigger points or acupuncture points with the intent of pain control.

acupuncture: An ancient Asian healing therapy employing the use of long, very fine needles; used in modern times as a method of pain control.

acute: Referring to brief exposure, sudden, of short duration, not chronic; sometimes used to mean severe.

acute mountain sickness (AMS): *See* altitude sickness.

acute otitis media: Inflammation of the middle ear.

acute respiratory disease: A life-threatening emergency in which O_2 levels drop and breathing becomes labored.

adaptation: Accommodation, to adjust to a stimulus.

addiction: A condition in which individuals cannot control their desire for alcohol, tobacco, food, exercise, or other activities.

Addison's disease: Chronic insufficiency of the adrenal cortex characterized by skin discoloration, anemia, weakness, and low blood pressure. Tuberculosis is the cause of approximately 20% of cases.

adduct: To move toward the midline in the frontal plane.

adduction (ADD): Movement toward the midline.

adenitis: Inflammation of the lymph nodes.

adenoidectomy: The surgical removal of the adenoids.

adenoids: Lymph tissue found in the superior aspect of the throat.

adenosine triphosphate (ATP): Adenine, ribose, and triphosphate; three phosphates that store energy that is released when ATP is split into ADP (diphosphate) or AMP (monophosphate).

adhesion: The union of tissue surfaces, also referring to the formation of scar tissue that often occurs following surgery.

adhesive capsulitis: Also known as "frozen shoulder"; a condition in which scarring occurs in the shoulder joint capsule; a complication of rotator cuff injury or bursitis.

adipose tissue: A term for "fatty tissue"; tissue composed mainly of fat cells.

adjuvant: From the Latin term adjuvans meaning "to help" or "to reach a goal"; adjuvant therapy is a form of treatment that increases the effect of a drug or increases the likelihood of a positive outcome.

adrenal gland: An endocrine organ that lies anteromedial to the kidneys and is responsible for production of glucocorticoid, mineralocorticoid, androgenic hormones, epinephrine, and norepinephrine.

adrenaline: Also known as epinephrine; a naturally occurring substance produced in the medulla of the adrenal gland; its release is part of the "fight-or-flight" response in which there is a dilation of blood vessels and an increase in heart rate and strength of contractions.

Adson's maneuver: A special test of the shoulder specifically for thoracic outlet syndrome. *See* Special Tests—Shoulder (Appendix 17).

adult-onset diabetes: *See* type II diabetes.

advance medical directives: Living will, durable power of attorney for health care, and health care proxy are examples of advance medical directives; instructions related to the treatment desires of an individual who cannot speak on his or her own behalf.

adverse effect: *See* adverse reaction.

adverse reaction: A negative or unwanted effect of a treatment.

aerobic training: Exercise that provides cardiovascular overload so as to develop functional capacity of the circulatory system and enhance aerobic capacity of specific muscles.

aesthesiometer: A device used to measure cutaneous sensitivity or the level of anesthesia. A two-point discriminator is an example of an aesthesiometer.

aetiology: *See* etiology.

affective disorder: A psychological condition in which the individual suffers extremes in moods and emotions; seasonal affective disorder (SAD) is an illness in which the individual is affected by the shorter days and lack of natural light during the fall and winter.

afferent: Conducting toward the center. In the case of nerves, conducting toward the brain, responsible for bringing sensory information to higher centers.

agenesis: The underdevelopment or nondevelopment of an organ or projection.

agonist: Muscle or muscle group responsible for a given joint motion. Its opposite is the antagonist.

AIDS: *See* acquired immunodeficiency syndrome.

AIDS-related complex: Symptoms related to HIV.

air embolism: Caused during surgery or from injury, it is the presence of air in the arteries that can cause a blockage.

airway obstruction: Anything that inhibits the passage of air to the lungs.

akinesia: Impaired body movement; absence of movement.

akinetic: Literally means "without movement"; refers to impaired, deficient, or lack of movement.

albinism: A disorder in which there is a reduction in melanin which is responsible for the pigment of hair, skin, and eye color.

albumin: A water-soluble protein responsible for the maintenance of plasma volume.

alcoholic cardiomyopathy: Heart damage or heart failure caused by the consumption of alcohol.

aldosterone: A hormone responsible for the regulation and balance of sodium and water in the body.

alimentary canal: The digestive tract.

alkalosis: A high pH; an abnormal condition in which there is a decrease in the normal acidity of the blood resulting from the accumulation of base or the depletion of acid. Can be caused by dehydration due to vomiting, hyperventilation, or high altitudes.

Allen's test: A special test of the shoulder used to assess thoracic outlet syndrome. *See* Special Tests—Shoulder (Appendix 17).

allergen: A substance that causes an allergic reaction.

allergic rhinitis: A reaction to a substance causing sneezing, runny nose, and sore eyes.

allograft: A transplant of tissue between allogeneic individuals (ie, a member of one's own species).

all-or-none response: The principle that describes the following: depolarization of a membrane requires a minimum intensity to reach threshold. Once threshold is met, depolarization occurs to the fullest extent. An increase in intensity has no increased effect.

alopecia: Baldness; alopecia areata is characterized by patchy bald spots; alopecia capitis totalis is total loss of hair.

alpha level: The probability of chance occurrence. The alpha level is chosen a priori (before beginning).

alprenolol: A beta-blocker used to treat high blood pressure, angina, and arrhythmias of the heart.

ALS: *See* amyotrophic lateral sclerosis.

alternating current (AC): A current that reverses its polarity; a current that crosses the isoelectric line; *see also* biphasic current.

alternative medicine: Holistic medicine; treatment methods not scientifically proven and generally not practiced in traditional medical facilities.

altitude sickness: An illness that affects nearly three-quarters of all people ascending to heights over 8000 feet. Symptoms include headache, dizziness, and nausea. The reduced air pressure can cause fluid to collect around the lungs and brain. If acclimatization does not occur, altitude illness can lead to a life-threatening condition.

alveolitis: Inflammation of the alveoli can progress to fibrosis or emphysema.

Alzheimer's disease: The most common form of dementia; it is a progressive disorder of the brain that first appears late in life and is characterized by memory loss, confusion, and a continued physical decline; marked by a degeneration of neurons in the cerebral cortex and the presence of beta-amyloid plaques. Named for Alois Alzheimer (1864-1915), a German neurologist who published a description of arteriosclerotic atrophy of the brain in 1894.

ambulation: The act of moving freely; walking.

ambulatory care: Outpatient care.

amenorrhea: The absence of the menstrual period for more than 3 months in women who had previously experienced menstruation and are not pregnant.

amine: A nitrogen compound derived from ammonia.

amino acid: A protein-building block.

amnesia: The loss of or impairment of memory: Anterograde is a loss of memory of events occurring after the injury; Retrograde is a loss of memory of events occurring prior to the injury.

amniocentesis: A procedure in which a small amount of amniotic fluid is removed from the mother's womb for testing of potential fetal disorders.

ampere (A): Unit of electrical current, abbreviated as amps; SI unit of electrical current, equal to the flow of 1 volt through or resistance of one ohm.

amplitude: Magnitude, intensity; depicted by the height of the waveform.

amyotrophic lateral sclerosis (ALS): Also known as Lou Gehrig's disease; a progressive disease of the motor neurons in which function is gradually lost.

anabolic steroid: A group of usually synthetic hormones that increase constructive metabolism. Anabolic steroids are frequently abused in sports that require strength and size.

anaerobic exercise: Activity in which the body incurs an oxygen debt; exercise occurring in the absence of oxygen.

analgesia: A state in which there is a reduction of or an inability to feel pain.

analgesic: A pharmacological agent designed to reduce pain.

analysis of covariance (ANCOVA): A statistical procedure designed to account for the influence of one or more variables that correlate.

analysis of variance (ANOVA): A statistical procedure used to establish whether a statistically significant difference exists between two or more samples.

anaphylactic shock: *See* anaphylaxis.

anaphylaxis: A histamine reaction to an allergen produced in response to injection. Can result in a severe systemic reaction including edema, circulatory failure, and death.

anastomosis: A communication between vessels or organs that are normally not connected; a surgical procedure in which a connection is made between healthy sections of the colon or rectum after a cancerous or diseased portion has been removed.

anatomical position: A reference position in which the body is upright, all joints are extended to the neutral position, and palms are facing forward.

anatomical snuffbox: A hollow on the radial aspect of the wrist when the thumb is extended caused by the tendons of the extensor pollicis longus and brevis. The name originates from the use of this space to hold powdered "snuff" tobacco.

anatomy: The study of body structure.

androgen: A male sex hormone that produces male sex characteristics.

anemia: Reduced hemoglobin; symptoms include fatigue, and decreased resistance to infection.

anesthesia: Decreased sensation caused by neurological dysfunction or pharmacological agent.

aneurysm: A bulge in the wall caused by localized dilatation of an artery, a vein, or the heart.

angina pectoris: Pain experienced in the chest, arms, or jaw because of a lack of oxygen to the heart muscle.

angioplasty: The use of surgery to make a damaged blood vessel function properly again; may involve widening or reconstructing the blood vessel.

Angiotensin-converting enzyme (ACE): A vasoconstricting peptide.

angle of pull (of a muscle): The angle formed by a longitudinal line through the bone from the axis and through the line of action (line of pull) of the muscle.

anisocoria: Unequal pupil size.

anisotropic: Having different mechanical properties depending upon direction of the load or force of application.

ankle mortise: The ankle joint; talocrural joint; the articulation between the tibia and the talus.

ankle-foot orthosis (AFO): A prosthetic for the foot or ankle; an AFO is commonly used for "drop-foot syndrome."

ankylosing spondylitis: Rheumatic disease of the synovial joints of the vertebrae. In severe cases, the spine becomes completely fused.

ankylosis: A disease process that results in the stiffening or fusion of a joint.

annulus fibrosis: The tough outer covering of a vertebral disk.

anode: The positive electrode. The electrode toward which negatively charged ions are attracted.

anomaly: A deviation from the norm.

anorexia nervosa: Most common in females, loss of appetite most commonly caused by an obsession to lose weight. Symptoms can be severe and can cause death.

anosmia: The loss of the sense of smell, often due to obstruction of the airway or injury to the olfactory nerve.

ANOVA: *See* analysis of variance.

anoxia: Decreased oxygen to the tissues, occurs frequently at high altitude.

antacid: A pharmacologic agent used to counteract the effects of hydrochloride acid released during digestion. Common agents include sodium bicarbonate, magnesium hydroxide, aluminum hydroxide, and calcium carbonate.

antagonist: The muscle or muscle group responsible for producing motions opposite of that being performed. The opposite of agonist.

anterior: Front, ventral.

anterior apprehension test: A special test of the shoulder to assess the anterior stability of the glenohumeral joint. *See* Special Tests—Shoulder (Appendix 17).

anterior cruciate ligament (ACL): A major ligament of the knee that prevents forward displacement of the tibia from the femur. The term cruciate literally means "to cross" and refers to the "crossing position" of the anterior and posterior cruciate ligaments. Females are two to eight times more likely to suffer ACL injury than males.

anterior draw (drawer) test: A special test of the knee to assess the continuity of the anterior cruciate ligament or of the ankle to assess the anterior talofibular, deltoid, and anterior tibiofibular ligaments. *See* Special Tests—Knee, and Ankle (Appendix 17).

anteroposterior: From anterior to posterior; from front to back.

anteversion: A forward displacement. An anteverted hip is characterized by increased medial rotation.

anthropometry: The science involved in measurement and comparison of the human body.

antibiotic: A pharmacologic agent used to treat infections by inhibiting the growth of microorganisms.

antibody: A protein that is part of the immune response that is produced by white blood cells in response to a foreign protein.

anticoagulant: A substance that hinders coagulation.

antiemetics: A pharmacologic agent used to treat nausea and vomiting.

antihistamine: A pharmacologic agent used to treat allergic reactions by inhibiting the effects of histamine.

antihypertensives: A pharmacologic agent used to treat high blood pressure.

anti-inflammatory: An agent used to reduce inflammation. *See* Appendix 18 for a list commonly used anti-inflammatory medications.

antioxidants: A substance that protects cells from oxygen free radicals.

antipruritic: A pharmacologic agent used to reduce itching.

antipsychotic: A pharmacologic agent used to treat severe mental disorders.

antipyretic: A pharmacologic agent used to reduce fever.

antiseptic: A bacteria-killing chemical used to prevent infections by its application on the skin.

anus: The opening at the distal end of the rectum.

aorta: The main artery leaving the heart responsible for supplying oxygenated blood to the body.

apex: The tip, or most superior portion, of a tissue.

aphasia: A disease of the left brain in which both speech and understanding of speech are affected.

aplasia: The complete or partial failure of any organ or tissue to grow.

aplastic anemia: A condition in which there is reduction in the number of red blood cells, white blood cells, and platelets.

Apley's compression: A special test of the knee used to assess the meniscus. *See* Special Tests—Knee (Appendix 17).

Apley's distraction: A special test of the knee used to differentiate between injuries to the meniscus and ligament injury. *See* Special tests—Knee (Appendix 17).

Apley's grind test: *See* Apley's compression.

Apley's scratch test: A special test of the shoulder used to determine range of motion. *See* Special Tests—Shoulder (Appendix 17).

apnea: A period where breathing stops.

aponeurosis: A fibrous sheath continuous with muscle fibers giving rise to the origin and insertion, in some cases becoming a tendon.

apophysis: A bony outgrowth; tubercles and tuberosities are examples of apophyses.

apophysitis: Inflammation of the apophysis, often at a point of tendinouos attachment.

apparent leg length: A leg length measurement taken from umbilicus to medial malleolus, useful only when true (real) leg length differences are negative. A positive test is indicative of pelvic obliquity.

appendectomy: The surgical removal of the appendix.

appendicitis: Acute or chronic inflammation of the appendix caused by blockage. Signs and symptoms include nauseau, fever, acute abdominal pain, particularly in the lower right quadrant, rebound tenderness over McBurney's point. Occasionally pain does not localize to lower right quadrant making diagnosis difficult. Surgery is usually required.

appendicular skeleton: The upper and lower extremities.

appendix: A small, finger-like projection of the large intestine.

apprehension test: A special test which by its nature causes the patient to become apprehensive or withdraw, especially when the sensation of dislocation is imminent; patella apprehension, anterior, posterior, and inferior (shoulder) apprehension.

approved clinical instructor (ACI): A certified athletic trainer who has successfully completed an ACI workshop conducted by the clinical instructor educator from the institution in which the ACI will be supervising athletic training students. In order to assess clinical proficiencies of a student enrolled in a Commission on Accreditation of Allied Health Education Programs (CAAHEP) accredited program, one must be an ACI.

approximate: To bring near, to place next to; the act of bringing the edges of a wound together.

approximation test: A special test used to assess sacroiliac dysfunction in which the patient is positioned side-lying, and the examiner applies a downward pressure of the iliac crest.

arch: A bony structure that resembles an arch and imparts elasticity or flexibility to it; the foot has four main arches. *See* lateral longitudinal arch, medial longitudinal arch, metatarsal arch, and transverse arch.

Arndt-Schultz principle: The amount of energy absorbed must be sufficient to stimulate the absorbing tissues or no reaction will occur.

arteriosclerosis: A disease in which there is progressive thickening and hardening of the walls of the arteries.

artery: A large blood vessel that carries oxygen-rich blood from the heart to the rest of the body.

arthokinematics: The study of joint movements.

arthralgia: Pain in a joint, not an inflammatory condition.

arthritis: Pain and stiffness characterized by inflammation of a joint.

arthrogram: Radiographs of a joint taken after injection of a contrasting medium (dye).

arthroplasty: The replacement of a joint or joint surfaces to restore the integrity and function of the joint.

arthroscopy: A surgical procedure performed through an endoscope.

arthrosis: Degenerative disorder of a joint.

articulate: Referring to an articulation, a joint.

articulation: A joint, a place where two or more bones are joined in such a way as to allow motion; *See also* uniarticulate, biarticulate, and multiarticulate.

artificial respiration: The act of providing ventilation for a person who has stopped breathing.

ascorbic acid: Vitamin C.

aseptic: Relating to a state of sterility, the absence of pathogenic organisms.

asphyxia: Suffocation; a situation in which an individual is unable to obtain adequate oxygen.

aspiration: The inspiration of fluid or foreign bodies into the lungs, such as with vomitus.

assumption of risk: A written statement signed by an athlete or his or her legal guardians stating that they are aware of the dangers inherent in participation in a particular sport and voluntarily accept the risk.

asthma: Also known as reactive airway disease; a narrowing of the airway due to swelling, spasm, or inflammation of the submucosa.

astigmatism: A condition of the eye in which the cornea is not exactly spherical; can often be corrected with lenses.

asymmetrical: Not the same, as in comparing one body area to its counterpart; the opposite of symmetrical.

asystole: The cessation of heartbeats.

ataxia: Jerky, uncoordinated movements of the limbs; an inability to move in a smooth coordinated fashion.

Ath: Abbreviation for "athlete."

atheroma: Atherosclerosis; a narrowing of the blood vessels caused by fatty deposits on the inner walls.

athlete's foot: *See* tinea pedis.

athletic pubalgia: Pain in the area of the pubic symphysis caused by muscle strain to one of the muscles that attach in the area such as the adductor longus, iliopsoas, rectus femoris, or rectus abdominus.

atrial fibrillation: An irregular heartbeat in which the atria beat "out of sync" and are ineffective in circulating blood.

atrium (atria-plural): The upper chambers of the heart.

atrophy: A wasting away of tissue; often used to describe loss of muscle tone.

attenuation: Loss of radiant energy due to reflection, refraction, or absorption; a decrease in intensity due to absorption into deeper tissues.

auditory nerve: *See* vestibulocochlear nerve.

auricle: External ear.

auricular hematoma: An inflammation of the external ear caused by repeated friction; common in the sport of wrestling. Commonly called cauliflower ear; also called hematoma auris; pinna hematoma.

auscultation: Listening to body sounds, usually with a stethoscope.

autism: Also known as Kanner's syndrome; self-absorption to the point of loss of reality characterized by repetitive and limited actions.

autogenic inhibition: A reflex activation of the antagonist and relaxation of the agonist caused by a sudden stretch.

autograft: A tissue or organ transferred from one part of a patient's body to another.

autoimmune disease: A disorder of the body in which the immune system is unable to distinguish between foreign material and that of itself and thus attacks its own otherwise healthy tissues.

automatic external defibrillator: An electric device designed to apply a "shock" to the heart with the intent of returning the fibrillating heart to normal sinus rhythm.

autonomic nervous system: The nervous system responsible for involuntary functions.

avascular: Lack of blood supply.

avascular necrosis: Death of a tissue due to lack of blood supply.

average current: The amount of current applied over a given time.

avulsion: A tear in which part of the structure is completely torn away.

axial skeleton: The skull, thorax, and spine.

axilla: Pertaining to the space inferior to the shoulder joint; under the arm; armpit.

axillary nerve: A branch of the brachial plexus; it is responsible for supplying the teres minor and deltoid muscles.

axonotmesis: Axonal compression injury in which the endoneural sheath remains intact and thus regeneration could occur.

B

Babinski's reflex/sign: A test for upper motor neuron lesion. The test is performed by running a blunt object on the plantar aspect of the foot starting at the calcaneus and moving upward in an arc toward the great toe. In the adult, a positive test is indicated by extension of the great toe and splaying of the lateral toes. This response is opposite in the infant.

bacitracin: An antibacterial ointment.

bacteremia: Bacteria found in the blood.

bacteriostatic: Halting the growth of bacteria.

bacterium: A small unicellular microorganism that multiplies asexually through cell division.

bacteriuria: Bacteria in the urine indicating infection of the bladder or kidneys.

Baker's cyst: A synovial fluid swelling in the popliteal space first reported in 1877 by William Morrant Baker, MD (1839-1896).

balance: A state of equilibrium; a constant state of motion in which attempts are made to keep the center of gravity well within the base of support; ability to maintain posture either statically or dynamically.

ballistic stretching: A stretching technique that uses momentum to force the tissue beyond its normal range of motion. Not synonomous with dynamic stretching.

bandage: A piece of cloth, gauze, or other material used to hold a dressing in place or to immobilize an injured body part.

Bankart's lesion: An avulsion of the anterior glenoid labrum caused by anterior dislocation.

barbituates: A group of drugs from barbituric acid that depress activity of the central nervous system; most are used as sleeping pills; a strong dependence may be developed and barbituates can be fatal when taken with alcohol.

barium enema: An enema used during an x-ray assessment of the large intestine and rectum to check for disease.

baroreceptors: A nerve ending responsible for sensing changes in pressure.

baroreflex: A reflex triggered by baroreceptors in an attempt to maintain pressure.

Barton's fracture: A fracture/dislocation of the distal radius.

basal cell carcinoma: Skin cancer found most commonly on the face, neck, and arms; caused by excessive exposure to sunlight.

basal metabolic rate: The rate at which energy is consumed at absolute rest.

baseline: A starting point that serves as a basis for comparison.

base of support: A kinesiology/biomechanics term that refers to the surface area of a body that is in contact with an external surface. For example, during single limb standing, the base of support is equal to the size of the foot.

basilar artery: Artery at the base of the brain. It later splits to form the two posterior cerebral arteries.

BCG vaccine: The vaccine for tuberculosis.

beam nonuniformity ration (BNR): The ratio of peak intensity to average intensity across an ultrasound head. A measure of the quality of the sound head. The closer the number is to one, the more even the beam.

beat: A waveform created by the combining of two waves from different circuits.

Becker's muscular dystrophy: A form of muscular dystrophy that starts later in life and advances more slowly; similar to Duschenne's; hereditary disease.

Bell's palsy: A unilateral paralysis of the face. The cause is unknown, and it usually resolves spontaneously. In some cases taste is affected and hearing becomes oversensitive.

Benazepril (Lotensin): An ACE inhibitor.

bends: *See* decompression sickness.

Benediction hand deformity: Also called Bishop's hand; a deformity caused by weakness of the thenar eminence, interossei, and two medial lumbricales due to ulnar nerve denervation. Flexion of fourth and fifth fingers is a sign.

benign tumor: A tumor that is not cancerous.

Bennett's fracture: A fracture/dislocation of the first metacarpal at the carpometacarpal joint.

beta blocker: A pharmacologic agent that reduces heart rate and the strength of the beat; it is used to treat high blood pressure and other heart diseases.

beta carotene: A substance found in orange fruits and vegetables that is converted to vitamin A.

beta (b) endorphin: A hormone naturally occurring in the brain having pain control properties similar to opiates.

biarticulate: Referring to the crossing of two joints. Example, the extensor carpi radialis longus crosses and performs a function at the elbow joint as well as the wrist.

bifid: A division into two lobes separated by a cleft.

bifocal: Glasses that are designed such that the upper portion of the lens restores distant vision while the lower portion of the lens restores near vision.

bilateral: Relating to both sides of the body.

bile: A substance produced by the liver responsible for the breakdown of fat and the removal of waste from the liver.

bile duct: The passageway from the liver to the gallbladder.

binging and purging: A characteristic behavior in individuals suffering from bulimia in which the individual eats to excess with gluttonous behavior and then either vomits or uses laxatives to rid him or herself of the food ingested.

bioavailability: A measurement of how fast and to what extent an active drug is metabolized and becomes "available" to the tissues in the system.

biochemistry: The science of the chemistry involved in living organisms.

bioequivalent: A drug that has the same effect on the body as another drug.

biofeedback: A means of giving a patient immediate feedback about bodily functions which are usually unconscious.

biomechanics: The study involving the knowledge and methods of mechanics that are applied to a human body.

biotransformation: A process in which substances in the body undergo chemical changes.

bipartate: Divided into two distinct parts.

biphasic current: A pulse that deviates from the iso-electric line first in one direction, then crosses the line and deviates in the other direction. *See also* monophasic current.

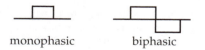

monophasic   biphasic

Examples of square monophasic
and square biphasic waveforms.

bipolar arrangement: An electrical stimulation pad placement that uses two active electrodes (pads) of equal size.

bipolar cells: A neuron that has two processes off the cell body.

Bishop's hand: *See* Benediction hand deformity.

bladder: Internal organ responsible for storage of urine.

blood borne pathogen: Infectious disease carried in the blood.

blood doping: A technique used by athletes to increase the oxygen-carrying ability of the blood by giving a blood transfusion (just before an event) of one's own blood that was previously withdrawn.

blood poisoning: *See* septicemia.

blood pressure (BP): Pressure created by the blood on the walls of the arteries. The normal average BP for an adult is a systolic pressure of 120 and diastolic pressure of 80 (120/80).

blow-out fracture: A fracture of the floor of the eye's orbit produced by a blow to the globe of the eye.

body composition: A measure of the ratio of body fat to lean body weight.

boil: An inflammation of the skin containing pus caused by staphylococcus bacteria which enters through a hair follicle or skin wound. See *also* furuncle.

bone marrow: The yellow fatty (or red at birth) tissue within the central medullary cavity of bone responsible for producing blood cells.

bone marrow transplant: A surgical procedure in which bone marrow is removed from a healthy area within the patient's body or from a donor and transplanted to a diseased area.

bone spur: An abnormal bony outgrowth in response to repeated trauma; a common site of bone spur formation is the calcaneus at the plantar fascia attachment.

Borg scale: A rating of perceived exertion.

Borg Scale of Perceived Exertion	
Numeric Rating of Exertion	Verbal Description of Exertion
6	None
7	Very, very light
8	
9	Very light
10	
11	Fairly light
12	
13	Somewhat hard
14	
15	Hard
16	
17	Very hard
18	
19	Very, very hard
20	

botulism: A type of food poisoning which occurs from ingestion of the neurotoxin clostridium botulinum, commonly occurring in improperly canned food.

bounce home test: A special test of the knee for meniscal injury. *See* Special Tests—Knee (Appendix 17).

boutonnière deformity: An injury to the extensor hood of the phalanges that causes flexion of the proximal interphalangeal and extension of the distal interphalangeal.

bowstring test: A special test for sciatic nerve involvement. *See* Special Tests—Spine (Appendix 17).

boxer's fracture: A fracture of the neck of a metacarpal (usually the fifth) with a volar displacement of the head of the metacarpal.

brachial plexus: A network of nerves made up of nerve roots (C4) C5-T1 that blend and divide to form a network and terminate as the peripheral nerves that supply the arm (axillary, musculocutaneous, median, ulnar, and radial nerves).

brachio: Arm.

brachy: Short.

bradycardia: An abnormally slow heart rate (less than 60 beats per minute).

bradykinin: A polypeptide hormone composed of a chain of nine amino acid residues formed during the inflammatory process causing vasodilation; responsible in part for the sensation of pain.

break test: A common method of assessing muscle strength. The patient is placed in mid range and the examiner attempts to "break" the contraction of the patient.

bronchitis: Inflammation of the mucous membranes of the bronchials.

bronchoconstrictor: A substance that causes the bronchial tubes to constrict or become smaller in diameter.

bronchodilator: A pharmacologic agent that dilates or increases the diameter of the bronchial tubes to improve breathing.

bronchospasm: A constriction or narrowing of the airway as a result of muscle contraction or inflammation; may be exercise induced (EIA—exercise-induced asthma), allergen induced, or caused by infection or other lung disease.

Brudzinski's sign: A variation of the straight leg raise in which neck flexion is combined with a straight leg raise. A positive sign of pain in the lumbar region or legs indicates nerve involvement.

bruise: *See* contusion.

bruxism: An involuntary action of grinding the teeth.

buccal: Referring to the cheek or mouth.

bulimia: A disorder in which the patient binges (ie, eats large amounts of food) and then purges the food by vomiting or using laxatives.

bunion: Localized inflammation and calcification of the first metatarsophalangeal joint either dorsal or medial; often associated with hallux valgus.

Bunnel-Littler test: A special test of the proximal interphalangeal joint to determine cause of tightness. *See* Special Tests—Hand/Wrist (Appendix 17).

burner: *See* neurapraxia.

bursa: A closed sac lined with synovial membrane containing fluid; acts as a cushion and lubricant and is found in areas subjected to friction.

bursitis: Inflammation of the bursa.

bursts: A series of electrical pulses delivered in packets or beats.

bypass: A shunt; a surgical technique in which a new path is created from which the flow of blood can "bypass" a blockage.

C

CAAHEP: *See* Commission of Accreditation of Allied Health Education Programs.

Café au lait macule: Areas of skin with increased melanin that appear with pale brown spots ranging from .5 - 8 inches in size and often disappear with age. Sometimes a sign of systemic diseases.

calcification: The process in which calcium salts are deposited in the tissue.

calcific tendonitis: Deposits of calcium in a tendon following chronic tendonitis.

calcium: Mineral that aids in nerve transmission, muscle contraction, blood clotting, heart functioning, and also works with enzymes.

callus: A thickening of the skin caused by repeated friction; new bone formation.

calor: Heat.

calorie: A unit of heat; the unit of measure for the amount of energy contained in food; the amount of heat required to raise 1 kg of water 1°C.

cancer: A term for malignant neoplasm.

candidiasis: An infection or disease caused by Candida albicans; occurs commonly in the vagina, and less commonly in the mouth or on the penis.

capacitance: The ability to store and separate an electric charge; the elasticity of a tissue.

capsular pattern: An abnormal movement pattern characteristic of each joint when there is capsular involvement.

captopril (Capoten): An ACE inhibitor.

carbohydrate: One of a group of compounds (mainly sugar and starch), made up of carbon, hydrogen, and oxygen; a main source of energy for the body that is eventually broken down to a simple sugar. Excess carbohydrate is stored in muscles and the liver as glycogen.

carbon dioxide: A colorless gas present in small amounts in the atmosphere and formed during metabolism; it is carried through the blood to the lungs where it is exhaled.

carbuncle: Formation of two or more boils coming together. Often caused by staphylococci; can result from shaving, chafing, or from dermatitis.

carcinogen: Any cancer-causing substance.

carcinoma: A cancer that occurs on epithelial tissue.

cardiac arrest: The sudden cessation of effective pumping action of the heart due to fibrillation or asystole.

cardinal planes: Three imaginary perpendicular reference planes that divide the body into equal halves. The saggital plane divides the body into left and right halves, the frontal or coronal plane divides the body into front and back halves, and the transverse plane divides the body into upper and lower halves.

cardiomyopathy: General term for any disease or abnormal condition of the heart muscle.

cardiopulmonary resuscitation (CPR): The administration of external cardiac compressions and artificial respiration to restore circulation.

cardiovascular system: The system responsible for circulating blood throughout the body including the heart and blood vessels.

carotene: An orange pigment (lipochrome) present in colored plants such as carrots; they include the precursor to the essential nutrient vitamin A.

carotid arteries: The two main arteries that carry blood to the head and neck (they further divide into the external and internal carotid arteries bilaterally).

carpals: Small bones of the hand (proximal row from lateral to medial: scaphoid, lunate, triquetrum, pisiform) (distal row from lateral to medial: trapezium, trapezoid, capitate, hamate).

carpal tunnel syndrome: One of the most common nerve entrapment syndromes. The median nerve becomes entrapped under the transverse carpal ligament. Characterized by pain and paresthesia in the median nerve distribution of the hand. Atrophy of the thenar eminence can occur.

carrying angle: The angle of the extended elbow (forearm supinated). The angle is determined by the intersection of imaginary lines through the long axis of the ulna and long axis of the humerus. Normal angle is 5-10° in males and 10-15° in females.

cartilage: An avascular connective tissue including hyaline, elastic, and fibrocartilage commonly found on bone ends, walls of the thorax, and tubular structures such as the ear canal and the airway. Most of the fetal skeleton is composed of cartilage and is later replaced by bone.

cast: A method of immobilization which often employs a plaster of paris or fiberglass shell.

catalysis: An increase in the rate of a chemical reaction induced by a catalyst.

catalyst: An enzyme that stimulates a chemical reaction to occur where it normally would be impossible, such as allowing a chemical reaction to occur at a temperature lower than it could usually occur.

cataract: Opacity or loss of transparency of the lens of the eye causing blurred vision.

catheter: A hollow tube-like device used to allow the passage of fluid.

catheterization: The insertion of a catheter or tube to permit influx or withdrawal of fluids.

cathode: The negative electrode.

cauda equina: The distal end of the spinal cord that forms the roots of the upper sacral nerves at the L1 level; resembles a "horse's tail."

cauda equina syndrome: Injury to the cauda equina often from disk lesion characterized by bilateral leg pain, diminished deep tendon reflexes, and bowel or bladder dysfunction. The patient with suspected cauda equina syndrome should be referred immediately to a physician.d

caudal: Toward the tail (or feet).

cauliflower ear: *See* auricular hematoma.

cauterization: The use of a cautery, a device that burns tissue with cryo-, thermo-, or electrotherapy to stop bleeding.

cavitation: Gaseous bubbles formed by the mechanical effect of therapeutic ultrasound.

cecum: The proximal end of the large intestine.

cell: The smallest living structure capable of independence; composed of a nucleus and a cell membrane made up of lipids and proteins capable of reproducing itself.

cellulitis: Inflammation of cellular connective tissue caused by bacterial infection often requiring the use of antibiotics.

center of balance: The point in the center between the feet or in the middle of the foot (in a single limb stance) in which 25% of the body weight falls in each of four quadrants measured two-dimensionally.

center of gravity: The central point about which the mass of an object is equally distributed.

center of pressure: Vertical ground reaction forces representing the center of the deviations measured three-dimensionally.

central biasing: Also known as descending inhibition; a theory of pain control in which pain is diminished through efferent impulses having left the higher centers to "block the gate" of pain transmission.

central nervous system: The part of the nervous system consisting of the brain and spinal cord.

centrifugal force: The force exerted radially outward on a body that is rotating about an axis.

centripetal force: The force exerted radially inward that is causing a body to travel in a circular path.

cephalad: Toward the head.

cerebellum: The largest part of the posterior brain; responsible for muscle tone, balance, and smooth coordinated movement, although not responsible for the initiation of voluntary motions.

cerebral palsy: A disorder commonly occurring before birth in which damage to the brain occurs causing weakness and uncoordinated movement of the limbs, and often affecting speech; spastic cerebral palsy is characterized by contractures which can progress to permanent deformity; uncontrolled writhing movements, called athetosis, are also common; causes include lack of oxygen, viral infection, and meningitis.

cerebrospinal fluid (CSF): A clear, watery fluid found in the subarachnoid space surrounding the brain and spinal column made up of glucose, salts, enzymes, and white blood cells.

cerebrovascular disease: Illness affecting the arteries that supply the brain; can lead to the formation of a blockage, resulting in a cerebrovascular accident, or stroke.

cerumen: Soft, waxy, brown secretion of the external auditory meatus.

cervical plexus: A network of nerves made up of the anterior branches of nerve roots C1-4 that blend and divide to form a network.

cervix: A neck-like structure at the distal end of the uterus.

cesarean section: A surgical procedure to remove the fetus from the womb through the abdominal wall; used when the health of the infant and/or mother would be at risk during natural childbirth.

C fiber: An afferent neuron responsible for carrying temperature and noxious stimuli; responsible for "slow pain."

chafing: A superficial skin wound caused by friction from skin rubbing skin.

chancre: A painless sore that occurs on the lips, eyelids, or genitals; a common sign of the sexually transmitted disease syphilis.

Charcot's syndrome: A disease of the spinal cord affecting one or more joints and ultimately resulting in a flail joint.

chemoreceptors: Afferent receptors sensitive to chemical changes.

chemotherapy: The use of chemical substances to treat infectious diseases and cancer.

Cheyne-Stokes breathing: An abnormal pattern of breathing in which the rate increases and decreases over a 1 minute period.

chickenpox: Varicella; a highly contagious disease transmitted by airborne herpes virus; characterized by fever and itchy red pimples; occurs most commonly during childhood.

chi square (P^2): A nonparametric statistical technique used to determine the significance between frequencies of nominal data.

Chlamydia: A bacterial illness that exists in the form of three species. The most common, Chlamydia trachomatis, is a sexually transmitted disease (STD) marked by penile discharge and painful urination in men, and symptoms ranging from none to vaginal or urethral discharge, lower abdominal pain, and acute pelvic inflammatory disease in women. It is the most common STD in the US with more than 4 million new cases each year.

cholecyst: The gallbladder.

cholecystectomy: The surgical removal of the gallbladder.

cholera: An acute epidemic disease caused by vibrio cholerae, causing severe diarrhea leading to dehydration and possibly death.

cholesterol: A fatty substance in blood and other tissues; important precursor of steroid hormones and bile salts; elevated levels associated with atheroma.

cholinergic: Nerve fibers that release acetylcholine as a neurotransmitter.

chondral: Cartilage.

chondral fracture: A fracture that also involves the articular cartilage of a joint.

chondritis: Inflammation of cartilage.

chondroma: A benign tumor in the cartilage.

chondromalacia: A degenerative condition in which there is a wearing away of the cartilage; on the posterior surface of the patella in chondromalacia patella.

chondrosarcoma: A malignant tumor that develops on the surface of a bone in the cartilage.

chronaxie: The phase duration required to cause an action potential when intensity is two times the rheobase.

chronic: Gradual onset; a disease or injury with a long duration.

cilia: Eyelash; a small, hair-like, motile structure found on the outside of some cells.

ciliary muscle: The muscle that controls the curvature of the lens of the eye.

CINAHL (Cumulative Index to Nursing and Allied Health Literature): An online resource for nursing and allied health professionals covering nursing, biomedicine, health sciences librarianship, consumer health, and 17 allied health disciplines. CINAHL indexes over 1200 nursing journals and other publications. It dates back to 1982.

circadian rhythm: The biological time clock.

circumduction: A circular movement made by a limb such as that made when one swings one's arms in a circle; the combined motions of flexion, extension, abduction, adduction.

cirrhosis of the liver: A progressive disease of the liver in which there is a gradual loss of liver function due to cell damage; there are many causes including long-term alcoholism.

Clancy test: A special test of the shoulder used to test for a SLAP lesion. *See* Special Test—Shoulder (Appendix 17).

Clark's sign: Also called patellar crunch or grind; a special test for chondromalacia of the patella performed by stabilizing the patella at the superior pole and asking the patient to contract the quadriceps. A positive test is indicated by pain. *See* Special Test—Knee (Appendix 17).

claudication: Ischemia most commonly of the triceps surae; a cramping pain in one or both legs while walking, which can cause limping.

claustrophobia: A fear of being in confined or crowded spaces.

clavicle: The horizontal s-shaped bone that runs from the sternum to the acromion process of the scapula; commonly referred to as the collarbone.

claw fingers: *See* clawhand.

clawfoot: Flexion contracture of the toes compounded by excessive pes cavus (high longitudinal arch).

clawhand: A hand deformity caused by injury to the median and ulnar nerves characterized by proximal phalanges that are hyperextended and middle and distal phalanges that are flexed.

claw toes: Characteristic extension of the MTP joints and flexion of the IP joints.

cleft lip: Harelip; a cleft palate that extends the entire palate and to the lip.

cleft palate: A fissure in the palate resulting from a birth defect in which the two sides of the palate fail to fuse together; can also occur with other birth defects such as cleft lip and partial deafness.

clinical instructor educator (CIE): A certified athletic trainer who has successfully completed the CIE training workshop and will train the approved clinical instructors for his or her academic program.

clinical trial: A research study involving a new drug or treatment.

clonus: Rhythmical limb movements such as those seen during a convulsive episode.

closed basket weave: Gibney technique; a taping procedure for ankle mediolateral instability.

closed (kinetic) chain: Referring to motion that takes place in which the proximal segments rotate about the fixed distal segment.

closed fracture: A bone break that does not break the skin.

closed packed position: A joint position when the bone ends are most congruent, joint surface contact is maximal and compressed.

closed reduction: The act of repositioning a displaced joint or bone without the need for surgery.

clubfoot: *See* talipes equinovarus.

coccyx: The distal bones of the spine which include four small fused bones forming a triangular shape at the base of the spine.

cochlea: The spiraled organ in the inner ear that picks up vibrations and transforms them into electrical signals that in turn are sent to the brain and interpreted as sound.

co-contraction: A muscular contraction in which both agonist and antagonist muscles contract simultaneously.

Codman's exercise: Pendulum exercises; passive range of motion exercises for the shoulder performed by the patient.

coefficient of friction: The ratio of the friction force to the perpendicular (normal) force pushing the two objects together.

colic: Severe waves of pain in the abdomen or urinary tract (in renal colic-kidney stones) often caused by a stone or intestinal infection.

colitis: Inflammation of the colon leading to abdominal pain, fever, and bloody diarrhea.

collateral: Accompanying, side by side; often used pertaining to the ligaments on either side of a joint, as in the knee including the medial (tibial) collateral and the lateral (fibular) collateral ligaments.

Colles' wrist fracture: A fracture of the distal radius in which there is a backward displacement below the fracture site.

colon: The middle portion of the large intestine, between the cecum and the rectum.

colonectomy: The complete or partial removal of the colon (large intestine).

colonoscopy: Visual examination of the colon using a long, flexible fiberoptic tube.

colostomy: A surgical procedure in which a stoma is formed by attaching the colon to the abdomen and thus making a new opening for feces to be excreted into a bag worn on the abdomen; *See also* ileostomy.

coma: A state of unconsciousness in which the individual cannot be aroused or can be aroused only minimally; the Glasgow coma scale is a means of "grading" the condition and takes into account whether the individual responds to verbal or painful stimuli.

comminuted fracture: A fracture in which there are many small pieces.

Commission of Accreditation of Allied Health Education Programs (CAAHEP): The accrediting body for several allied health professions, including entry-level athletic training education programs.

communicable disease: A disease that can be spread from one individual to another.

compartment syndrome: A condition in which inflammation causes increased pressure in a compartment and thus increased pressure on the nerves and blood supply that are contained in the compartment. Occurs commonly in the compartments of the lower leg, especially the anterior compartment. Onset of compartment syndrome can be acute or chronic.

compliance: The extent to which the patient adheres to medical advice.

compound fracture: An open fracture; a fracture in which the bone ends protrude through the skin.

compression fracture: A fracture in which a bone is broken due to compressive forces.

compression test: Special test of the cervical spine for nerve root compression. *See* Special Tests—Spine (Appendix 17).

computed tomography scanning: CT, CAT scan; a radiological technique for producing cross-sectional images of the body that are then analyzed with a computer.

concave: A surface that is curved inward.

concave-convex rule: In joint mobilization, the rule related to movement of a concave bone on a convex bone describing accessory motion that is in the same direction as the physiological motion. *See also* convex-concave rule.

concentric contraction: A muscular contraction in which the muscle is shortening.

concussion: An injury to the brain caused by a blow to the head in which there are disturbances in the electrical activity in the brain; symptoms include headache, nausea, loss of consciousness, memory loss, and other neuropsychological impairment. Common grading systems and return to play criteria can be found in Appendix 9.

conduction: A method of heat transfer through direct contact with an object of a different temperature.

confidence interval: A pair of numbers on either end of a range from a sample that has a particular probability of including the population parameters.

congenital: Describing that which was present at the time of birth.

congestive heart failure: A condition in which the heart is ineffective at circulating blood and results in fluid accumulation and congestion of the lungs.

conjunctiva: The clear membrane that covers the front of the eye and lines the eyelids.

conjunctivitis: Also known as pink eye; inflammation of the conjunctiva caused by allergy, chemical reaction, or virus, in which case it will quickly spread to the other eye.

connective tissue: Strong fibrous tissue that connects and supports body structures including tendon, ligaments, cartilage, bone, adipose tissue, and elastic structures.

constipation: A condition in which there are incomplete or infrequent bowel movements and feces are dry and hard.

continuing education units (CEU): NATABOC Athletic trainers are required to complete 80 CEUs every 3 years.

continuous passive motion machine (CPMM): A device used to provide passive movement of a joint; usually used following surgery to reduce loss of motion.

contracture: Muscle shortening due to muscle spasm or fibrosis.

contraindication: A treatment not recommended or inadvisable due to the current condition.

contralateral: Denoting the opposite side.

contrecoup injury: Lesion within the skull opposite to the side in which the blow occurred.

contusion: Internal damage to the tissue as a result of a blunt trauma resulting in discoloration.

convection: A method of heat transfer in which heat is transferred indirectly through medium such as air or liquid.

convex: A surface that is curved outward; *See also* convex-concave rule.

convex-concave rule: In joint mobilization, the rule related to movement of a convex bone on a concave bone describing accessory motion that is in the direction opposite the physiological motion. *See also* concave-convex rule.

convulsions: Waves of involuntary muscular contractions and relaxations.

core stability: A fine line between mobility and stability, it is functional stability of the trunk with appropriate biomechanical alignment between the pelvis and shoulder girdle and efficient, coordinated neuromuscular recruitment of the trunk.

corn: A thickened callus that forms over a bony prominence, commonly in the toes.

cornea: Continuous with the conjunctiva, it is the clear, anterior one-sixth of the eye, serving as the main refractory structure of the eye focusing light on the retina.

coronal plane: Also known as frontal plane; divides the body into dorsal and ventral or anterior and posterior parts. Motions that take place in this plane include abduction/adduction, radial/ulnar deviation, and lateral flexion of the trunk and head.

corticosteroids: Any steroid synthesized by the adrenal cortex; synthetic corticosteroids are used for the powerful anti-inflammatory effect created by suppression of the immune system.

coryza: Inflammation of the mucous membrane of the nasal airway caused by the common cold or allergies.

cosine law: Electromagnetic radiations travel in a straight line, therefore the ideal position is at a right angle to the target tissue.

costo: Denoting the ribs.

costochondral: The junction of the ribs and the cartilage between the ribs and the sternum.

costoclavicular: The articulation of the ribs and clavicle.

costoclavicular syndrome test: A special test of the shoulder to assess thoracic outlet syndrome. *See* Special Tests—Shoulder (Appendix 17).

ounterirritant: An agent that creates a mild irritation and acts as an analgesic. Examples include heat, cold, and superficial analgesics.

coupling medium: A substance used to reduce impedance and facilitate conductivity.

coxa: Hip.

coxalgia: Hip pain.

coxa plana: A degenerative disease of the capital femoral epiphysis. *See also* Legg-Calvé-Perthes disease.

coxa valgus: A condition in which the angle between the axis of the femoral neck and the long axis of the femoral shaft is greater than 135 degrees.

coxa vara: A condition in which the angle between the axis of the femoral neck and the long axis of the femoral shaft is less than 135 degrees.

cranial: Relating to the head.

creatine: A substance that combines with phosphate to form creatine phosphate (phosphocreatine) a high-energy phosphate released during anaerobic muscular activity. Recently taken as a supplement. Side effects and effects of long-term use are not fully understood.

creatinine: A urinary waste product of phosphocreatine metabolism produced by the kidneys. The normal creatinine level is 1.2 mg/dL.

crepitation: Fine crackling sensation such as that felt when palpating over a fracture site.

crepitus: A grating sensation in a joint or tendon due to swelling or degenerative changes.

criterion referenced tests: Tests which have a predetermined standard of performance.

Crohn's disease: Ulcerative colitis; inflammatory disease affecting the distal end of the ileum in which there is thickening and ulcerations. Treatment includes antibiotics, immunosuppressive drugs, and in some cases removal of the affected part of the intestine.

cross-arm adduction test: *See* cross-over impingement test.

cross-over impingement test: A special test of the shoulder to assess impingement. *See* Special Tests—Shoulder (Appendix 17).

crural index: The ratio of upper leg length to total leg length.

cryokinetics: Application of cold prior to or simultaneous to an exercise regime.

cryotherapy: Treatment involving the use of cold and ice.

CT scanning: *See* computed tomography scanning.

cubital tunnel: A tunnel formed by the ulna, ulnar collateral ligament, and the flexor carpi ulnaris muscle through which the ulnar nerve passes.

cubital tunnel syndrome: Compression of the ulnar nerve as it passes through the cubital tunnel.

cubital valgus: A condition in which the carrying angle of the elbow is greater than 15°.

cubital varus: A condition in which the carrying angle of the elbow is less than 5-10°. A gunstock deformity is a severe case of cubital varus.

culture: The propagation of cells or microorganisms in a laboratory setting.

current density: Amount of electrical current per given area.

curvilinear: The path of movement along a curved line.

cyanosis: A bluish discoloration of the skin beginning around the lips, caused by reduced oxygen levels.

cyclist's knee: *See* iliotibial band friction syndrome; also known as runner's knee.

cyst: Abnormal closed sac filled with fluid and lined with epithelial tissue.

cystectomy: Surgical removal of the bladder; a length of the small intestine can be used to form a "new bladder," or in some cases a urostomy is necessary.

cystic fibrosis: A genetic disorder affecting the exocrine glands resulting in production of a thick mucous which can obstruct the lungs, pancreas, or intestinal glands; infection is common; treatment is aimed at reducing bronchial stress and preventing infection.

cystoscopy: Examination of the bladder and urethra using a cystoscope.

D

Daily Adjustable Progressive Resistance Exercise (DAPRE): Described by Ken Knight, this is a protocol involving increased resistance exercise 6 days per week in which the following procedure is followed: the first set consists of 10 repetitions at 50%, followed by the second set consisting of 6 repetitions at 75%, followed by the third set consisting of as many repetitions as possible at 100%, followed by the fourth set of as many as possible adjusted from the first set as described next. The fourth set is adjusted based on the number of repetitions performed in the third as follows: 0 to 2 repetitions, decrease weight and redo set; 3 to 4 repetitions, decrease by 5 pounds; 5 to 7 repetitions, use the same weight; 8 to 12 repetitions, increase by 5 to 10 pounds; 13+ repetitions, increase 10 to 15 pounds.

deafferentation: A loss or reduction of afferent input.

debridement: The removal of foreign material and dead tissue from an open wound.

decay: Tissue death.

deceleration: Decrease in velocity per unit of time (meters per second per second-m/s^2). For example, -1 m/s^2 means that velocity is decreased by 1 m/s every second.

decerabrate (rigidity): Abnormal posture indicating brain stem injury; extension and adduction of the upper extremity joints; and extension, internal rotation, and plantar flexion in the lower extremity.

decompression sickness: "The bends"; a common injury in scuba diving caused by ascending too quickly; gas bubbles are formed in the body's tissues.

deconditioning: A period in which an athlete loses his or her fitness level.

decorticate (rigidity): Abnormal posture indicating injury above the brainstem; flexion and adduction of the upper extremity joints; extension, internal rotation, and plantar flexion in the lower extremity.

decubitus: Lying down.

deep: Underneath, further from the surface.

deep tendon reflex: An involuntary muscular contraction controlled by the reflex arc and caused by a sudden stretch imposed on a tendon.

deep-vein thrombophlebitis: A thrombosis associated with inflammation of a vein wall.

deep-vein thrombosis: A blood clot commonly occurring in the veins of lower leg, causing pain.

defecation: The act of moving the bowels.

defibrillation: The use of an electric shock in an attempt to re-synchronize the defibrillating heart.

deficit: A decrease in functional capacity as when compared bilaterally or to the norm.

degenerative arthritis: *See* osteoarthritis.

degrees: A unit of measure for range of motion in which a complete circle is divided into 360 equal parts; a unit of measure for temperature.

degrees of freedom: The number of variables that are free to vary when restrictions are set.

dehydration: A condition in which there is a severe loss of fluid (water) from the body.

dementia: A gradual decline in mental ability; Alzheimer's disease is the most commonly known form of dementia.

dendrite: A branching process of a neuron that conducts impulses toward the soma (cell body).

density: Mass or weight per unit volume.

dental caries: Cavities or tooth decay.

deoxyribonucleic acid (DNA): The genetic make-up of all living organisms.

dependent variable: Dependent measure; in research, it is the variable that is measured.

depolarization: The act of neutralizing a cell membrane's resting potential.

depression: A lowering or downward movement.

de Quervain's disease: A tenosynovitis of the extensor pollicus brevis and abductor pollicus longus caused by repetitive motion.

dermabrasion: A procedure in which the surface of skin is removed through abrasion, commonly with a sanding device; a common treatment for scarring or the removal of tattoos.

dermatitis: Inflammation of the skin.

dermatome: A sensory area of the skin supplied by a particular nerve root.

dermis: The deep layer of skin.

descriptive statistics: The statistics used to describe a set of data.

desensitization: To lessen sensitivity by nerve block or otherwise interfering with nerve conduction.

deviate: To vary from the norm.

deviated septum: Displacement of the ethmoid and/or vomar bones causing disruption of continuity of the nasal septum.

deviation score: The difference of a score from the mean.

dextrose: Glucose.

diabetes insipidus: A rare metabolic condition characterized by increased urine production treated with the hormone vasopressin.

diabetes mellitus: A common form of diabetes in which glucose is not oxidized due to the lack of insulin production from the pancreas. Control is maintained by dietary intake and the use of insulin. *See* insulin shock and diabetic coma.

diabetic coma: A condition in which a person who suffers from diabetes loses consciousness due to hyperglycemia. Diabetes mellitus is a chronic metabolic disorder in which the pancreas does not produce insulin

(Type I) or there is an increased resistance to insulin or reduction in production (Type II). In patients with known diabetes, diabetic coma is most commonly caused by failure to take insulin. *See also* insulin shock.

diagnosis: A process of disease identification through its signs and symptoms.

dialysis: A process in which blood is removed from an artery and enters a dialyzer (filtering machine); the blood is filtered and returns through a vein. This procedure is used to treat kidney failure, to remove waste products, maintain acid-base balance, and remove excess fluid from the body.

diapedesis: Emigration; the passage of blood cells through the intact capillary wall.

diaphragm: A large muscle found between the abdomen and chest cavity responsible for breathing. When the diaphragm contracts, pressure in the chest decreases and forces air in the airway into the lungs. When the diaphragm relaxes, air is expelled through the airway. Also, a thin, latex, dome-shaped apparatus used as a method of contraception.

diaphysis: The shaft of a long bone.

diarthrodial: A type of joint in which opposing bones move freely. Hinge and ball & socket are types of diarthrodial joints.

diastole: The relaxation period of the heart between two contractions at which time the heart chamber fills with blood.

diastolic pressure: The blood pressure measured when the heart is in diastole (relaxation phase in which the ventricle fills with blood); the normal systolic pressure in an adult is 120 mmHg, normal diastolic pressure in an adult is 80 mmHg, recorded as 120/80 mmHg.

diathermy: A deep heating modality from the electromagnetic spectrum that uses high frequency electromagnetic energy. Shortwave diathermy has wavelengths ranging from 11 to 22 m and operates at a frequency of approximately 13 to 27 MHz; microwave diathermy has wavelengths ranging from 12 to 70 cm and operates at a frequency of approximately 430 to 2,450 MHz.

differential diagnosis: A process of diagnosing an injury or illness which shares common signs and symptoms with other conditions and thus, must be ruled out.

diplegia: Bilateral paralysis, often more severe in the legs.

diplopia: Double vision.

direct current: An electrical current that does not alternate polarity; does not cross the isoelectric line.

direct service: Treatment or other services provided directly to one or more patients by a practitioner.

disk injury: Herniated disk; bulging disk; injury to the annulus fibrosis (outer covering) of the vertebral disk in which a portion of disk material protrudes and places pressure on a nerve root, causing numbness, tingling, weakness, impaired deep tendon reflexes, and, most commonly, pain along the nerve distribution. The severity of injury depends on the amount of pressure applied by the disk material as well as secondary swelling. Protrusion, prolapse, extrusion, and sequestration are common disk injuries.

dislocation: A third-degree sprain in which two or more bones are displaced at the joint. A partial, incomplete or an immediate, spontaneous relocation is referred to as a subluxation.

dispersive electrode: A large "not active" electrode used to complete the electrical circuit. Due to its size, current density is low and thus the dispersive electrode is not an "active" electrode. The use of a dispersive pad constitutes a monopolar pad placement.

distal: Further away from the point of origin; further from the beginning; further from the trunk.

distention: Stretching of the bladder or stomach; swelling; enlargement.

distraction: To pull apart; a special test in which a joint is distracted (pulled apart) causing a reduction of symptoms.

diuretic: A pharmacologic agent designed to increase the amount of water in the urine thereby removing excess water from the body; commonly used to treat fluid retention and hypertension.

diverticula: Small sacs on the inner lining of the intestine.

diverticulitis: Inflammation of diverticula.

domain: A specific performance area. The 12 domains in athletic training education include "risk management and injury prevention," "pathology of injuries and illnesses," "assessment and evaluation," "acute care of injuries and illnesses," "pharmacology," "therapeutic modalities," "therapeutic exercise," "general medical conditions," "nutritional aspects," "psychosocial intervention and referral," "health care administration," and "professional development and responsibility."

dominant gene: A powerful gene in that whenever it is present, it always produces its effect.

don: "To put on" as in clothing.

dorsal: Back, posterior.

dorsal: Pertaining to the back; dorsum.

dorsiflexion: Flexion of the foot toward the shin; to bring the "toes up."

Down syndrome: Trisomy 21, a genetic disorder in which there are three number 21 chromosomes, causing moderate to severe mental handicap and a characteristic appearance of slanted eyes, small ears, flat nose bridge, and short stature.

downward rotation: Movement of the scapula about an anteroposterior axis such that the glenoid fossa turns in a downward direction.

dressing: A wound covering often held in place by a bandage.

drop arm test: A special test of the shoulder for rotator cuff injury. *See* Special Tests—Shoulder (Appendix 17).

drop foot syndrome: A condition caused by weakness of the dorsiflexors in which the individual is unable to dorsiflex and thus, unable to support the foot during the swing phase of the gait; therefore, the foot "drops;" commonly caused by anterior compartment syndrome of the lower leg.

Duchenne's Muscular Dystrophy (MD): *See* muscular dystrophy.

Dupuytren's contracture: An abnormal fusion of the flexor tendon to the skin of the third and fourth fingers, causing a flexion contracture.

dura: The thick, outermost covering of the brain and spinal cord.

duration: Length of time; in modalities it refers to treatment time; the measure of the length of time of an electromagnetic wave (ie, the phase duration of the pulse is 200 microseconds).

duty cycle: A relationship of the on time to the off time over a specified period. A treatment in which there is a 5 msec on time and 5 msec off time has a 50% duty cycle.

dynamic flexibility: The available range of motion during active (dynamic) motion.

dynamic splint: A splint that is designed to provide continuous passive or active assisted stretch.

dynamic stretching: A gradual, controlled increase in stretch and speed of motion taken to the limits of ROM.

dynamometer: A device used to record muscular force.

dysmenorrhea: Painful menstruation.

dysplasia: Excessive tissue development; monostotic fibrous dysplasia and polysotic fibrous dysplasia are conditions in which bone, commonly in the legs, is replaced by fibrous tissue causing pain and difficulty walking.

dyspnea: Difficulty breathing.

E

eccentric contraction: A muscular contraction which takes place during muscular lengthening.

ecchymosis: Discoloration caused by extravasation of blood into the tissues.

echocardiogram: An ultrasound image of the heart.

ectomorph: A somatotype (ie, body type) characterized by being tall and thin.

ectopic: Located in an abnormal position.

ectopic pregnancy: A condition in which the fertilized ovum is deposited outside the uterus, most commonly in the fallopian tubes; occurs in 1 out of 150 pregnancies.

eczema: Inflammation of the skin characterized by itching and scales; cause is often unknown, can occur due to allergies.

edema: Accumulation of fluid in the body; in injury, caused by the effects of inflammation.

effective radiating area (ERA): The area of the sound head (ultrasound) which has been deemed to effectively deliver ultrasound. For example, an ultrasound head that measures 5 cm^2 may only have an ERA of 4.7 cm^2. In order to be considered in the ERA, 5% of the initial intensity must be measurable at a depth of 5 cm.

efferent: Conducting away from the center. In the case of nerves, conducting away from the brain, responsible for conducting impulses from the brain to the organs or tissues.

efficacy: The capability of having the desired effect.

effleurage: A type of therapeutic massage involving a rhythmical motion in one direction with the intent of increasing blood flow.

effusion: Excess blood or fluid in the tissues.

Ehlers-Danlos syndrome: A genetic disorder of connective tissue characterized by hypermobility of the joints, delicate skin that bruises easily, subcutaneous cysts, and visceral deformity.

EKG: A graphical representation of the electrical activity of the heart. The first wave, the "P" wave, indicates depolarization of the atria. The "Q, R, and S" waves indicated depolarization of the ventricle, and the "T" wave indicates ventricular repolarization.

elasticity: The ability to return to its original shape once tension is released.

elastic limit: Yield point; the point on a stress strain curve at which further stress will cause permanent deformation.

elastic modulus: The ratio of stress to strain (ie, the slope of the line).

elbow flexion test: A special test of the elbow to assess ulnar nerve entrapment. *See* Special Tests—Elbow (Appendix 17).

elective: Referring to a treatment or procedure that is not necessary and can be "elected" as a form of treatment by the patient; often not covered by medical insurance.

electrical impedance: Resistance, the opposition to electron flow.

electrocardiogram (ECG or EKG): An instrument that measures the electrical impulses of the heartbeat.

electroencephalography: A process of assessing brain activity by recording the brain's electrical impulses.

electrogoniometer: An electrical device used to measure range of motion.

electromagnetic field: Forms of energy emanating from an electrical source; an electrical field created by the lines of force between the two poles.

electromagnetic spectrum: A means of displaying the relationship between various forms of energy by placing them along a continuum in order by wavelength, including cosmic and gamma rays, visible light, infrared modalities, and electrical stimulating modalities.

elevation: To raise up; upward movement of the scapula.

Ely's: A special test of the hip to assess hip flexion contracture, specifically the rectus femoris. *See* Special Tests—Hip (Appendix 17).

embolism: The blockage caused by an embolus.

embolus: Material in the blood, such as a blood clot, fat, air, bacteria, amniotic fluid, bone marrow, cholesterol, etc, that circulates in the blood from one place to another and becomes lodged.

embryo: An animal in the early stages of development; in humans it refers to the first 8 weeks following fertilization.

EMG: Electromyogram. A graphical representation of muscular activity in response to electrical stimulation.

empty can test (supraspinatus test): A special test of the shoulder to assess the rotator cuff. *See* Special Tests—Shoulder (Appendix 17).

EMS: Abbreviation for "emergency medical services" or "electrical muscle stimulation." For this reason, NMES (neuromuscular electrical stimulation) is preferred.

endemic: Describes a disease that tends to be present within a certain group of people.

end feel: The normal or abnormal sensation or resistance felt by the examiner at the end of a passive range of motion. *See* Appendix 15.

endocrine gland: A hormone-secreting gland that secretes directly into the blood. The pituitary, thyroid, parathyroid, adrenal, ovaries, and testes are examples of endocrine glands.

endogenous: Arising from inside of the body.

endogenous opioids: A hormone naturally occurring in the brain having pain control properties similar to opiates.

endometriosis: The presence of endometrium in other areas of the pelvis causing severe pain lasting several days each month.

endometrium: The membrane lining the uterus.

endomorph: A somatotype (ie, body type) characterized by being short and overweight.

endorphin: One of a group of naturally occurring chemicals produced in the brain exhibiting strong pain relieving properties similar to that of opiates.

endoscope: A lighted instrument with an optical system used to transmit images from the inside of a body cavity.

endothelium: A thin layer of tissue cells that line the heart, blood, and lymphatic vessels.

endpoint: *See* end feel.

endurance: The ability to perform activity for an extended period of time without fatigue; the ability to bear pain, adversity, and stress.

energy: The capacity to perform work.

enkephalin: A protein neurotransmitter that inhibits the release of substance P, thereby blocking the transmission of noxious stimuli from first order to second order neurons.

enteritis: Inflammation of the small intestine.

enuresis: Bed wetting.

enzyme: A protein that speeds up biological reactions.

epicondylitis: Inflammation of the epicondyle at the origin of the wrist extensors (lateral epicondylitis) or wrist flexors (medial epicondylitis).

epidemic: A sudden outbreak of an illness that spreads rapidly.

epidemiology: The study of illness, disease, or injury for the purpose of discovering its cause and preventing future cases.

epidermis: The outermost layer of skin.

epidural anesthesia: A procedure to block pain in which a pain-relieving pharmacologic agent is injected into the epidural space around the spinal cord to block sensation to the abdomen and lower extremities; this procedure is commonly used during childbirth or for lower extremity surgery.

epidural hematoma: Bleeding in the brain above the dura matter, usually arterial bleeding with rapid onset of symptoms. Compare to subdural hematoma.

epilepsy: A disorder of unknown cause affecting the nervous system in which there is abnormal electrical activity in the brain causing petit mal and grand mal seizures; epilepsy is controlled with anticonvulsant drugs such as dilantin.

epinephrine: Also known as adrenaline; a hormone secreted by the adrenal glands in response to stress or fear; responsible for the "fight-or-flight" response in which there is an increase in heart rate, metabolism, and improved breathing.

epiphysis: The end of a long bone, separated from the diaphysis by the metaphysis to allow for bone growth and eventual fusion to the diaphysis.

epiphysitis: Inflammation of the epiphysis, most commonly in infants, affecting the hip, shoulder, and knee.

epitaxis: Nosebleed.

epithelium: Tissue covering the external surface of the body and lining the hollow organs.

Epstein-Barr virus: A virus that causes mononucleosis; spread by mucous secretions.

equinus deformity: A congenital deformity of the foot in which there is a contracture of the plantar flexors of the foot; gait is marked by toe walking.

Erb palsy: A birth defect in which there is a lesion to the upper trunk of the brachial plexus or the nerve roots from C5-6 causing weakness or paralysis of the deltoid, biceps, brachialis, and brachioradialis.

ergometer: Mechanical device used to assess the amount of work done. A bicycle is an example of a lower body ergometer (LBE).

ergonomics: The study of man in his work surroundings; the "application of scientific information concerning humans to the design of objects, systems and environment for human use." (The Ergonomic Society)

erysipelas: Fever and rash caused by streptococci bacteria.

erythema: Redness of the skin.

erythrocyte: Red blood cell.

erythroplakia: A precursor to cancer characterized by red patches in the mucous membranes of the mouth, throat, or larynx; tobacco users have increased risk.

esophageal reflux: *See* gastroesophageal reflux.

esophageal spasm: A contraction of the smooth muscle of the esophagus that causes difficulty swallowing.

esophagus: The portion of the digestive tract connecting the throat to the stomach.

estrogen: One of a group of steroid hormones synthesized mainly in the ovaries responsible for female sexual development.

estrogen replacement therapy: A treatment using the synthetic form of estrogen to treat amenorrhea, symptoms of menopause, to aid in the prevention of osteoporosis and heart disease in women, and cancer of the prostate in men.

ethics: A system of morality, of right and wrong.

etiology: The study of the causes or origins of disease or injury.

euthanasia: The act of ending the life of a terminally ill patient who requests to die.

evaluation: The interpretation of a test.

evaporation: A method of heat transfer by which a liquid is converted into a gas.

eversion: The movement of the plantar aspect of the foot laterally, or away from the midline.

exacerbation: To increase the severit;, to aggravate.

excision: The surgical removal of tissue.

exogenous: Arising from outside of the body.

exostosis: A bony outgrowth.

expectorant: A pharmacological agent used to "break up" phlegm by promoting coughing.

extension: A movement of a joint such that the angle formed by the two bones increases.

external rotation: To turn a body segment about its long axis so as to turn the anterior aspect of the segment toward the outside or laterally; also called lateral or outward rotation.

exteroreceptor: An afferent receptor in the skin or mucous membrane that responds to stimuli from outside the body.

extracorporeal lithotripsy: A noninvasive procedure to break down a kidney stone through the use of shock waves.

extradural anesthesia: *See* epidural anesthesia.

extravasation: Fluid (commonly blood) that has escaped through outlying tisses.

extrinsic: A term used to describe something originating from outside an organ or body segment; opposite of intrinsic.

exudate: Accumulation of fluid with a high concentration of proteins, cells, or debris.

F

FABRE test (or FABER): Test for the hip involving Flexion, Abduction, and External Rotation; also known as FABER or Patrick's test. *See* Special Tests—Hip (Appendix 17).

face validity: The extent to which a measure seems to test the outcome based on your instincts (face value). The weakest measure of construct validity.

facet joint syndrome: A painful inflammation of the facet joints of the vertebrae.

facial nerve: The seventh cranial nerve; regulates facial movements, sensation, and taste on the anterior portion of the tongue. *See* Appendix 8.

facial palsy: Unilateral paralysis of the facial muscles caused by inflammation of a nerve.

factor analysis: A statistical procedure that analyzes the relationship of multiple variables and their contribution to the entire set of variables.

faint: Syncope; loss of consciousness due to insufficient blood flow to the brain.

false negative: A situation in which a patient is found not to have a disease or condition, due to a faulty test procedure, when in fact they do have the disease.

false positive: A situation in which a patient is found to have a disease or condition, due to a faulty test procedure, when in fact they do not have the disease.

familial: A term used to describe conditions that tend to "run in the family."

fartlek training: "Fartlek" from the Swedish word for "speed play"; a type of interval training that uses varied speeds and terrains.

fascia: A band of strong connective tissue that binds structures together.

fasciitis: Inflammation of the fascia covering the muscles.

fast twitch fiber: *See* type II fiber.

fatigue: The inability to continue an exercise.

fat soluble vitamins: Vitamins A, D, E, and K.

fatty acid: An important component of lipids; a long hydrocarbon chain with an even number of carbon atoms.

FDA: Food and Drug Administration.

felon: Infection of the palmer side (pulp) of the finger which becomes inflamed and swollen and often filled with pus. Most commonly caused by staphylococcus; can occur from small nick, hangnail, splinter, or incision to the finger tip. Generally requires minor surgery.

female athlete triad: A common combination of anorexia (or bulimia), amenorrhea, and osteoporosis.

femoral artery: The main artery that supplies blood to the legs, found most superficially in the femoral triangle.

femoral nerve: Nerve of the anterior thigh that innervates the quadriceps; it passes through the femoral triangle.

femoral nerve test: A traction test in which the patient is side-lying with affected side up and neck slightly flexed. The examiner extends the hip approximately 15 degrees with the knee extended followed by a flexing of the knee. Pain radiating into the anterior thigh is a positive test.

femoral triangle: A triangular shaped area located in the anterior, proximal thigh bordered by the inguinal ligament and the sartorius and adductor longus muscles. The femoral nerve and artery pass through this triangle.

femur: The long bone of the thigh.

fibrillation: A rapid and irregular rhythm of the heart muscle fibers causing a lack of synchrony such that there is an inability to efficiently pump blood.

fibrin: The final product in the formation of a blood clot. The mesh-like substance is the product of fibrinogen.

fibrinogen: A substance found in the blood that when acted upon by thrombin produces fibrin.

fibroadenoma: A benign tumor of the breast.

fibrocartilage: A dense type of cartilage found between the vertebra and at the pubic symphysis.

fibrocystic breast disease: The most common cause of benign breast lumps.

fibroid: A benign uterine tumor.

fibroma: A benign tumor found in connective tissue.

fibrosis: Abnormal scar formation in connective tissue.

Finkelstein's test: A special test of the wrist to test for the presence of de Quervain's. *See* Special Tests—Hand/Wrist (Appendix 17).

first-class lever: A type of machine in which the axis is between the motive and resistive forces. Examples include pliers, scissors, and a teeter-totter. The advantage of a first-class lever depends on the relative length of the moment arms of the motive and resistive forces. In the human body there are few first-class levers. One example, however, is the action of the gastroc/soleus unit (motive force) at the ankle joint (axis) during a toe-standing motion (ground reaction force is the resistive).

first-order neuron: Afferent neurons in the periphery.

first ray: The first phalanx and first metatarsal joint of the foot.

fissure: A groove or cleft-like defect.

fistula: An abnormal opening from an organ or structure.

fitness: A measure of one's strength, flexibility, and endurance.

fixation: A stabilization technique.

flaccidity: Decreased muscle tone.

flatulence: Abdominal or intestinal gas expelled through the anus.

flexibility: Mobility; the range of motion about a joint.

flexion (FLEX): The movement at a joint in which the segments of a joint are brought toward each other; a movement of a joint such that the angle formed by the two bones decreases.

flu: *See* influenza.

fluidotherapy: A form of thermotherapy involving the use of very fine, dry particles flowing about the injured part.

fluoride: A mineral that helps prevent tooth decay.

fluoroscopy: An x-ray device that allows images to be seen directly on a fluorescent screen without the need for developing film.

folliculitis: Boils or blisters caused by the inflammation of hair follicles due to a bacterial infection.

foramen: An opening or hole in a bone.

force: A push or pull that causes or tends to cause a change in shape or motion and is measured in pounds or Newtons.

force arm: The perpendicular distance from the axis of rotation to the line of action of the force.

forefoot valgus: A midtarsal eversion deviation with neutral subtalar joint. During weight-bearing, the midtarsal joint is supinated and the lateral aspect of the forefoot strikes the ground. Contributes to pes cavus.

forefoot varus: A midtarsal inversion deviation with neutral subtalar joint. During weight-bearing, the midtarsal joint is pronated bringing the 1st metatarsal toward the ground. Contributes to pes planus.

forward head: A posture characterized by positioning the head in an anterior position such that the neck exhibits a marked extension in the area of C4-C6. Often accompanies kyphosis and is a common cause of chronic neck and shoulder pain.

free nerve endings: Nociceptors; nerve endings that are particularly sensitive to mechanical, thermal, and chemical noxious stimuli.

frequency: The number of cycles, pulse repetitions per unit of time. Measured in hertz (Hz).

frequency distribution curve: The organization of test scores into intervals.

friction: The force resisting the "sliding" of one object past another.

friction massage: A type of therapeutic massage used to loosen adhesions, reduce spasm, and assist in absorption of edema. Small circular motions with the thumb, finger, or palm of hand are used to move the superficial tissues over the underlying tissues.

frontal plane: Divides the body into dorsal and ventral or anterior and posterior parts. Motions that take place in this plane include abduction/adduction, radial/ulnar deviation, and lateral flexion of the trunk and head.

frostbite: Freezing or partial freezing of human tissue such as when exposed to prolonged or extreme cold.

functional assessment: Testing procedures that mimic the neuromuscular demands of various sports skills.

functional exercises: Exercises that require the patient to execute various activities that call upon the neuromuscular system to perform similarly to those activities involved in sport.

functional leg length: An assessment of leg length by comparing the height of the anterior superior iliac spine (ASIS) in the standing patient.

functional position: The act of placing a limb or joint in the position most appropriate or most used.

functional progression: A series of sport-specific and graduated exercises designed with the intent of returning the individual safely and efficiently to full participation.

furuncle: An inflammation of the skin containing pus caused by staphylococcus bacteria, which enters through a hair follicle or skin wound.

furunculosis: A condition resulting form the presense of boils (furuncles).

G

Gaenslen's: A special test of the sacroiliac joint. *See* Special Tests—Hip (Appendix 17).

gait: Walking pattern.

galactose: A form of sugar created from the breakdown of lactose.

gallbladder: A small organ (sac) just inferior to the liver, in which bile is stored.

gallstone: A hard mass made up of cholesterol, bile pigments, and/or calcium salts that is found in the gallbladder.

Galvanic electrical stimulation: Direct current electrical stimulation, named for Luigi Galvani (1737-1798), who was an Italian physician and physicist known for his electrical stimulation experiments of frog nerves and muscles.

Galveston Orientation and Amnesia Test (GOAT): A test that measures early recovery of memory and orientation to person, place, and time.

ganglion: A cyst-like structure that often forms in a tendon, commonly found in the wrist. An enlarged area in the posterior sensory root of a spinal nerve.

gangrene: Tissue death due to lack of blood supply.

gapping test: A special test of the sacroiliac joint. *See* Special Tests—Hip (Appendix 17).

gastrectomy: The surgical removal of the stomach or part of the stomach.

gastric acid: The digestive acid in the stomach that breaks down proteins.

gastric ulcer: A peptic ulcer.

gastrin: A hormone produced in the pyloric region of the stomach that stimulates the production of gastric acid.

gastritis: Inflammation of the lining of the mucous membrane of the stomach; causes may include virus, bacteria, alcohol, and drugs.

gastroenteritis: Inflammation of the stomach and intestines.

gastroesophageal reflux: Also called esophageal reflux. A condition in which gastric acid reenters the esophagus causing heartburn and esophagitis.

gate control theory: A theory of pain control based on the assumption that painful stimuli carried by Ad and C afferent nerves and sensory stimuli carried by Ab afferent nerves converge upon the dorsal horn in the substantia gelatinosa (SG). The larger Ab impulses travel faster and reach the SG and act to close the gate to the painful stimuli.

gene: The basic unit of DNA that controls the formation of a single polypeptide chain which determines the biochemical makeup of the proteins, rate of protein production, and the integration of protein into the cell structure.

generic drug: A drug name that indicates the class or type of compound.

gene therapy: An experimental medical procedure in which diseased or disease-causing genes are replaced by healthy ones.

genital herpes: Inflammation of the skin caused by the herpes simplex virus characterized by small blisters; transmitted through sexual contact.

genu: A sudden anatomical turn as in flexion; in orthopedics the term is used to denote the knee.

genu recurvatum: Hyperextending knees.

genu valgum: Literally means "knee turned outward," referring to the deformity in which the tibia is angled outward. The common term is "knock knees."

genu varum: Literally means "knee turned inward," referring to the deformity in which the tibia is angled inward. The common term is "bow-legged."

Gibney: Closed basket weave; a taping procedure for ankle mediolateral instability.

gingivectomy: Surgical removal of diseased tissue of the gums.

gingivitis: Inflammation of the gums. Common causes include poor dental hygiene, build-up of plaque, poorly fitting appliances, scurvy.

gland: An organ responsible for secreting fluid either through specialized ducts (exocrine glands) or directly into the bloodstream (endocrine glands).

Glasgow coma scale: A means of assessing level of consciousness based on motor, verbal, and eye opening response.

Glasgow Coma Scale		
Eyes	spontaneously	4
	to verbal command	3
	to pain	2
	no response	1
Verbal	oriented and converses	5
	disoriented and converses	4
	inappropriate	3
	incomprehensible	2
	no response	1
Motor	obeys verbal commands	6
	localizes painful stimulus	5
	normal flexion withdrawal	4
	decorticate posture	3
	decerebrate posture	2
	no response	1
	TOTAL	3-15

glaucoma: A disease of the eye in which increasing pressure in the eye can cause an eventual loss of sight if pressure is not controlled.

glenohumeral: The shoulder joint; the articulation between the head of the humerus and the glenoid fossa of the scapula.

gliding joint: A diarthrodial joint in which motion is created when the articular surfaces glide upon each other without axial motion.

glossopharyngeal nerve: Cranial nerve IX, responsible for swallowing and taste. *See* Appendix 8.

glucagon: A hormone produced by the pancreas that increases blood sugar by converting stored carbohydrates (glycogen) into glucose, thus having the opposite effect of insulin.

glucose: A simple sugar, it is the main source of energy for the body and the sole source of energy for the brain; glucose is stored in the body as glycogen.

glucose tolerance test: A test for diabetes mellitus in which the concentration of sugar in the blood and urine are tested over time in response to the intake of a known amount of glucose following a period of fasting.

glycogen: The stored form of glucose; stored in muscles and in the liver.

glycosuria: The presence of glucose in the urine.

Godfrey's sign: A special test for posterior cruciate ligament instability. *See* Special Tests—Knee (Appendix 17).

goiter: Swelling in the throat, in particular the thyroid gland; causes include lack of iodine in the diet, or hyperthyroidism.

golfer's elbow: *See* medial epicondylitis.

golgi tendon organ (GTO): Mechanoreceptor that is sensitive to changes in length and tension. When the GTO is stimulated, it causes a reflex relaxation (autogenic inhibition) of the antagonist muscle(s).

gonadotropic hormones: One of the hormones released by the pituitary gland that stimulate activity in the ovaries and testicles.

goniometer: A protractor-like device used to measure joint angle.

gonorrhea: A common sexually transmitted disease caused by the bacterium *Neisseria gonorrhoeae* and characterized by painful urination and discharge from the penis or vagina.

gout: A disease that affects the joints, caused by excess uric acid in the joints; may also affect the kidneys.

graft: A procedure in which healthy tissue is used to replace diseased or damaged tissue.

grand mal: A convulsive type of seizure.

Graves' disease: An autoimmune disease that causes hyperthyroidism and a subsequent goiter and characteristic bulging eyes.

gravity: A motive force that is always present and acts on the center of gravity of every object. Acceleration caused by the force of gravity is -9.8 m/s^2 or 32 ft/s^2. In other words, an object that is dropped from a building will be traveling at a velocity of -9.8 m/s^2 exactly 1 second after it is released and 19.6 m/s^2 exactly 2 seconds after it is released, etc.

ground fault interrupters (GFI): An electrical safety device that will cause the electrical current to shut off if it detects leakage of current.

ground reaction force: The equal and opposite force applied by the ground in response to the force applied to the ground as in walking, running, jumping, etc.

Guillain-Barré syndrome: A disease affecting the peripheral nervous system causing inflammation, weakness, and loss of sensation in the arms and legs; appears 10 to 20 days after a respiratory infection.

gunstock deformity: Cubitus varus caused by humeral condylar fracture.

gynecomastia: Enlarged breast tissue in males. Can occur at birth, at onset of puberty, and again around the 5th decade of life.

H

half-value thickness: The depth of a tissue or substance at which the intensity of a beam of radiation will reach half of its original value.

halitosis: Bad breath.

hallucination: The perception of something that is not really there, for example, "seeing or hearing things."

hallux: Great toe.

hallux rigidus: A restriction of flexion/extension of the first metatarsophalangeal joint.

hallux valgus: Bunion; angling inward of the great toe.

Halstead's maneuver: A special test of the shoulder for thoracic outlet syndrome. *See* Special Tests—Shoulder (Appendix 17).

hammer toe: A flexion deformity of the proximal inter-phalangeal joint of the toe, commonly the second toe.

hangman's fracture: A fracture of the pedicle of C2, some-times accompanied by anterior dislocation of the body of C2.

harelip: *See* cleft lip.

Hawkins-Kennedy impingement test: A special test of the shoulder for impingement. *See* Special Tests—Shoulder (Appendix 17).

HDL: *See* high-density lipoprotein.

heartburn: Caused by acid reflux, a recurrent burning sen-sation in the chest and throat.

heart murmur: An abnormal heart sound heard during auscultation.

heart rate: The rate at which the heart "beats" in 1 minute.

heat cramps: Muscle spasm brought on by prolonged exposure to heat, humidity, and/or the presence of dehydration.

heat exhaustion: Heat illness brought on by prolonged exposure to heat, humidity, and/or the presence of dehydration. Symptoms include rapid pulse, pale skin, profuse sweating, and increased body temperature (rectal) to 102°F. Treatment includes immediate removal from heat and rapid oral and intravenous rehydration.

heat illness: One of the many forms of illness brought on by dehydration and/or exercising in excessive temperatures and humidity levels.

heat rash: Prickly heat; a local rash brought on by prolonged exposure to heat.

heat stroke: A serious, life-threatening form of heat illness brought on by prolonged exposure to heat, humidity, and/or the presence of dehydration. Symptoms include loss of consciousness; shallow breathing; rapid pulse; red, hot skin; mild to no sweating; and core temperature (rectal) of 106°F or higher. Treatment includes immediate removal from heat and rapid oral and intravenous rehydration.

heel counter: The portion of a shoe that encloses the calcaneus and provides rearfoot stabilization.

heel strike: The point at which the heel makes contact with the ground following the swing phase of the walking or running cycle.

Heimlich maneuver: A first aid technique used to dislodge a foreign object from a choking person's airway.

hemarthrosis: Bleeding and swelling in a joint.

hematemesis: Vomiting of blood.

hematocrit: The percentage of red blood cells in the total blood volume.

hematoma: The formation of a blood clot within the tissue, initially may appear as swelling.

hematuria: Blood in the urine.

hemiparesis: *See* hemiplegia.

hemiplegia: Paralysis affecting one side of the body. The face and upper extremity are often more affected.

hemodialysis: *See* dialysis.

hemoglobin: An iron-containing porphyrin responsible for the pigment in red blood cells and for carrying oxygen throughout the body.

hemolysis: The normal process in which red blood cells are broken down in the spleen.

hemophilia: An inherited disorder in which the blood clots too slowly leading to prolonged bleeding; caused by a lack of antihemophilic factor (factor VIII).

hemopoietic: Related to the formation of blood cells.

hemorrhage: Bleeding.

hemorrhoid: A distended vein at the opening of the anus caused by straining.

hemostasis: The normal clotting process which controls bleeding.

hemothorax: Blood in the pleural cavity between the chest wall and the lungs.

hepatic: Pertaining to the liver.

hepatitis: Inflammation of the liver; causes include alcohol abuse, drug use, viral infection, or poisons. Symptoms include fever, headache, nausea, and general weakness. Hepatitis A (infectious hepatitis) is transmitted through contaminated food or water; hepatitis B and C (serum hepatitis) are transmitted through sexual contact or contact with bodily fluids; hepatitis D is a form of hepatitis that only appears when hepatitis B virus is already present.

Herb's palsy: *See* Erb's palsy.

hereditary: Passing a genetic trait from parent to offspring.

hernia: Protrusion of an organ or tissue through an opening as in a weakening in the surrounding wall.

herniated vertebral disk: A condition in which the annulus fibrosis of the vertebral disc fails and the nucleus bulges or extrudes through the outer wall placing pressure on the spinal nerve roots. *See* disk injury.

herpes simplex: The simple form of the herpes virus, characterized by blisters on the face, mouth, or genitals.

herpes zoster: "Shingles;" characterized by pain along the distribution of a nerve; *See also* chicken pox.

hertz (Hz): The SI unit of frequency.

hiccup: Involuntary spasm of the diaphragm along with the closing of the glottis, producing a "hiccup" sound.

high-density lipoprotein (HDL): Considered to be the "good cholesterol"; a specific protein in the blood thought to remove cholesterol, thereby protecting against heart disease.

high-voltage current: A type of electrical nerve stimulation that uses voltage greater than 150 volts with pulses of very short duration, commonly a twin peak pulse.

Hill-Sachs lesion: A defect in the posterior articular cartilage of the humeral head found after anterior dislocation of the shoulder.

HIPAA: The Health Insurance Portability and Accountability Act of 1996 is a privacy provision that applies to health information created or maintained by health care providers. It seeks to ensure privacy of individually identifiable healthcare information.

HIPS: Systematic evaluation procedure consisting of History, Inspection, Palpation, and Special Tests. *See also* HOPS (observation instead of inspection).

hirsutism: Excessive growth of hair in unusual places, especially in women.

histamine: A compound associated with mast cells that is released during allergic reactions, causes dilation of blood vessels and contraction of smooth muscle, especially the lungs, causing a narrowing of the airway.

histamine blocker: A drug that inhibits the action of histamine; H1 blocker is used to treat inflammation; H2 blocker is used to block the production of stomach acid to treat peptic ulcers.

HIV: *See* human immunodeficiency virus.

hives: The common term for an itchy rash resulting from an allergic reaction.

Hodgkin's disease: A malignant disease of the lymph nodes and spleen; symptoms include enlarged lymph nodes, fever, loss of appetite, and weight loss.

Hoffman's reflex (digital): Special tests for upper motor neuron lesion in which the examiner "flicks" the distal phalanx of the first, second, or third finger. A reflex flexion of the thumb or adjacent finger (not flicked) is a positive sign.

Homan's sign: A special test for deep vein thrombophlebitis. The patient's foot is passively dorsiflexed while the knee is extended. *See* Special Tests—Knee and Leg (Appendix 17).

homeostasis: The tendency of a system to maintain stability.

homogeneity of covariance: Equality of correlation among three or more repeated measures taken on the same subjects.

homogeneity of variance: Equality of variance among two or more measures.

Hoover's test: A special test used to test for malingering. *See* Special Tests—Spine (Appendix 17).

HOPS: Systematic evaluation procedure consisting of History, Observation, Palpation, and Special Tests. *See also* HIPS (inspection instead of observation).

hordeolum: *See* stye.

horizontal: Parallel to the floor, perpendicular to a vertical line.

horizontal abduction: Movement away from the midline in the transverse plane. When the limb is abducted to 90 degrees and then moved horizontally away from the midline or toward the back it is called horizontal abduction. When the limb is flexed to 90 degrees and then moved in the same direction it is called horizontal extension.

horizontal adduction: Movement toward the midline in the transverse plane. When the limb is abducted to 90 degrees and then moved horizontally toward the midline or toward the front it is called horizontal adduction. When the limb is flexed to 90 degrees and then moved in the same direction it is called horizontal flexion.

horizontal extension: An extension movement that takes place in the transverse (horizontal) plane. *See also* horizontal abduction.

horizontal flexion: A flexion movement that takes place in the transverse (horizontal) plane. *See also* horizontal adduction.

hormone: A substance produced by an endocrine gland and released into the blood stream; acts to control or modify an organ or tissue.

Hughston test: *See* jerk test of Hughston.

human immunodeficiency virus (HIV): The virus that causes AIDS; contracted through sexual intercourse or contact with infected blood.

human papilloma virus (HPV): A virus that causes various human warts to the hands, feet, genitals, and anus; some are associated with cancer.

hunting response: The vasodilation that follows the initial vasoconstriction after the application of cold.

hydrocele: Swelling of the scrotum.

hydrocephalus: "Water on the brain;" an abnormal increase in cerebrospinal fluid around the brain.

hydrocortisone: A corticosteroid used to treat inflammation and allergies.

hydrotherapy: The therapeutic use of water.

hyper: A prefix denoting an increase, excessive, above, or more than.

hyperabduction syndrome: Symptoms of thoracic outlet syndrome caused by abduction of the arm.

hyperemia: A collection of excess blood.

hyperextension: Extreme extension; beyond normal extension.

hyperglycemia: Abnormally high glucose levels caused by undiagnosed or improperly treated diabetes mellitus.

hyperhidrosis: Excessive sweating.

hypermobility: An abnormal increase in range of motion; excessive joint play; commonly referred to as "double-jointed." A sign of Marfan's and Ehlers-Danlos syndromes.

hyperopia: Far-sightedness.

hyperparathyroidism: Increased calcium levels in the blood and decreased calcium levels in bones caused by overactivity of the parathyroid glands.

hyperplasia: Hypertrophy; an increase in growth of cells.

hyperpnea: Hyperventilation.

hyperreflexia: An abnormal increase in normal reflex response.

hypertension: High blood pressure.

hyperthermia: Elevated body temperature; *See* heat illness.

hyperthyroidism: Overactivity of the thyroid gland.

hypertonic (hypertonus): An abnormal increase in muscle tone; a solution that has increased osmotic pressure.

hypertrophic cardiomyopathy: A thickening of the cardiac muscle walls causing arterial obstruction and leading to mitral valve prolapse and possible aortic rupture.

hypertrophy: Increase in the size of a tissue due to an enlargement of the cells rather than multiplication of cells.

hyperventilation: Rapid breathing characterized by a reduction in CO_2 in the blood.

hyphema: A collection of blood in the anterior chamber of the eye.

hypo: A prefix denoting a decrease or lack of; under; below.

hypoglossal nerve: Cranial nerve XII, responsible for swallowing and movements of the tongue. *See* Appendix 8.

hypoglycemia: A decrease in blood glucose; occurs in diabetes patients with an inadequate intake of carbohydrates.

hypoplasia: The failure of a tissue or organ to fully develop.

hyporeflexia: Decreased reflex.

hypotension: Abnormally low blood pressure.

hypothenar: The medial side of the "heel of the hand."

hypothermia: Body temperature below 95°F caused by prolonged exposure to cold temperatures.

hypothyroidism: Underactivity of the thyroid gland; symptoms include decreased heart rate, weight gain, and apathy.

hypotonic (hypertonus): An abnormal decrease in muscle tone; a solution that has decreased osmotic pressure.

hypoventilation: Abnormally slow breathing rate.

hypovolemic shock: Shock induced by loss of fluid, commonly due to excessive internal or external bleeding. Also may be caused by excessive vomiting or diarrhea.

hypoxia: Decrease in oxygen supplied to the tissues.

hysterectomy: The surgical excision of the uterus.

iatrogenic: Referring to an illness or medical condition caused as a direct result of the treatment; a complication of a medical treatment.

idiopathic: Unknown cause.

Ila: Inferiolateral angle (of the sacrum).

ileostomy: A medical procedure whereby the ileum is brought through the abdominal wall to form a new opening (stoma).

ileum: The distal end of the small intestine leading to the large intestine.

iliotibial band (ITB) friction syndrome: A chronic injury caused by the friction created when the ITB rubs over the lateral femoral epicondyle. Common in running and cycling athletes. Also known as runner's knee. *See* Special Tests—Hip (Appendix 17).

ilium: One of the two large, flat, dish-shaped bones of the hip.

immune: A resistance to disease; not susceptible to a particular disease; possessing the antibodies to fight off a particular antigen.

immune system: The system including the thymus, spleen, and lymph nodes that protects the body from disease organisms and foreign substances.

immunodeficiency: May be genetic or acquired; characterized by a decreased ability to launch an effective immune response.

immunology: The study of the immune system.

immunostimulant: A drug that increases the immune system and improves the body's ability to fight disease.

immunosuppressant: A drug that inhibits the immune system and thus prevents the body from attacking itself; commonly used to prevent rejection following organ transplant.

impedance (active electrode): The resistance in a tissue to the flow of electrical current.

impetigo: A bacterial skin infection that is highly contagious; caused by staphylococcal and sometimes streptococcal, occurs around the nose and mouth and rapidly spreads into patches of crusty pustules.

implant: A device or tissue surgically placed in the body.

impotence: A condition in which a male suffers from the inability to acquire or maintain an erection of the penis.

incision: A cut or wound caused by a sharp straight object such as in surgery.

incisor: One of the eight front teeth.

incontinence: Inability to control the release of urine or feces.

independent variable: A variable controlled by the research design that may have influence on other variables (ie, the dependent measure).

Index Medicus: An extensive medical index of the National Library of Medicine in which journal information is listed by subject, author, title, key words, journal, year, and country of publication.

indigestion: A feeling of discomfort following eating caused by abnormal digestion or ingestion of irritable foods.

inertia: The resistance to changes in movement.

infarction: The death of an organ due to loss of blood flow usually caused by a blood clot.

infection: Invasion of the body by a pathogen.

inferential: A type of research design in which inferences are made.

inferior: Below, lower than.

inflammation: The immediate response following injury that may be caused by mechanical, thermal, chemical, or infection; signs and symptoms include redness (rubor), pain (dolor), swelling (tumor), heat (calor), loss of function (functio laesa).

inflammatory bowel disease: Crohn's disease or ulcerative colitis.

inflammatory joint disease: Swelling, redness, and pain around a joint; any type of arthritis.

influenza: A highly contagious viral infection affecting the respiratory system. Symptoms include weakness, cough, fever, and muscle aches.

informed consent: A process by which a subject or patient is fully informed of the possible benefits and dangers of a medical procedure or participation in a research study and voluntarily agrees to participate.

infrared: The part of the electromagnetic spectra just before visible light; infrared modalities include ice, cold packs, cold whirlpool, vapocoolant sprays, warm whirlpool, hydroculator packs, and paraffin.

ingestion: To eat or drink; to take by mouth.

ingrown toenail: A painful condition in which the edge of the nail grows into the skin, commonly in one of the distal corners; caused by improper clipping of the toenail.

inguinal hernia: Protrusion of an organ or tissue through an opening at the inguinal canal.

inhaler: A pharmacologic agent in the form of a gas or vapor that is breathed into the lungs to treat conditions of the lungs, especially asthma.

inherited: A trait that is passed from parent to child.

injection: The act of using a syringe to inject a drug.

innominate bone: The lateral half of the pelvis consisting of the ilium, ishium, and pubis.

insemination: Injection of semen into the vagina.

insertion: A place of muscular attachment to a bone. The insertion is the attachment on the moveable segment or the attachment furthest from the midline of the trunk.

in situ: "In place;" refers to a disease that has remained localized.

insomnia: Inability or difficulty sleeping.

instability: In orthopedic assessment, the state of a joint when the ligaments fail to support it.

insulin: A protein hormone produced in the pancreas important in regulating the absorption of glucose and thus controlling blood sugar levels; diabetes is the inability to produce the hormone or adequate amounts of the hormone and is treated with insulin injections.

insulin shock: A condition in which a person with diabetes takes too much insulin or takes the required amount but fails to eat. This situation results in a serious hypoglycemic condition and is life-threatening.

intensity: (In modalities) Amplitude; the rate at which energy is delivered.

interclass correlation (interclass reliability coefficient): An estimation of reliability that uses correlational procedures.

interferential: A type of electrical stimulation in which two channels of differing frequencies "interfere" with each other, causing periods of constructive and destructive interference, creating a "beat" frequency equal to the difference between the two frequencies (ie, channel A at a frequency of 4000 and channel B at a frequency of 4010 produce a beat frequency of 10 Hz).

intermittent compression: A form of mechanical therapy in which compression is alternately increased and decreased to assist the pumping action of the lymphatic system. Intermittent compression is used to treat lymphedema and other edemas.

internal fixation: A method of stabilizing a fracture with surgically placed screws, rods, and plates.

internal rotation: A rotation movement so as to turn the anterior aspect of the segment toward the inside or medially; medial rotation; inward rotation.

interneuron: A neuron in the central nervous system that acts as a link between two neurons.

interoreceptor: An afferent receptor in the skin or mucous membrane that responds to stimuli from within the body such as tissue tension or chemical changes.

interosseous membrane: The connective tissue between two or more bones.

interstitial: A space between tissues or body parts.

interstitial cystitis: Inflammation of the lining of the bladder.

intertrigo: Skin chafing.

intervertebral disks: A broad, flexible, fibrocartilagenous disk found between each vertebrae that functions to connect the vertebrae, provide cushioning, and promote movement between vertebrae; made up of a fibrous outer layer called the annulus fibrosis and a gel-like inner layer called the nucleus pulposis; *See also* herniated disk.

intestine: The continuation of the alimentary canal, from the stomach to the anus, divided first into the small intestine (duodenum, jejunum, ileum) and then the large intestine (cecum, vermiform appendix, colon, rectum).

intraclass correlation (ICC; intraclass reliability coefficient): An estimation of reliability that uses analysis of variance.

intractable: A disease that does not respond to treatment.

intramedullary rod: A long metal rod that is placed into the medulla of a fractured bone.

intraocular pressure: The pressure created by fluid levels in the eye.

intravenous: Pertaining to the inside of a vein.

intrinsic: A term used to describe something originating from and located within an organ or body segment; opposite of extrinsic.

invasive: A medical procedure in which an instrument is introduced into the body tissues through the skin or body orifice; a tumor or microorganism that spreads throughout body tissues.

inversion: Of the foot, motion of the foot so as to turn the sole of the foot inward.

inversion stress test: The inversion force of the talar tilt test, a test in which the ankle is inverted to assess the lateral ligaments of the ankle.

in vitro: Literally means "in glass;" a test or procedure that is carried out in a laboratory setting, ie, not in a living being; the opposite of in vivo.

in vivo: Literally means "in the living body;" a test or procedure that occurs in a living being.

involuntary: Independent to volition; in treatment or research circumstances, a situation in which the individual did not provide informed consent.

inward rotation: A rotation movement so as to turn the anterior aspect of the segment toward the inside or medially; medial rotation; internal rotation.

iodine: A nonmetallic element with several uses including as a contrast or stain for testing, as a topical antiseptic, and as a treatment for thyroid disease.

ion: Electrically charged atom.

iontophoresis: The use of electrical stimulation (direct current) to drive ions to deeper tissues.

ipsilateral: Denoting the same side.

iris: The colored part of the eye, responsible for the regulation of light that enters the eye by the muscular ring formed around the pupil.

iron: A metallic element that occurs in the important biological substances such as the heme of hemoglobin, myoglobin, and certain other enzymes; iron deficiency leads to anemia; meat and liver are good dietary sources of iron; the recommended daily intake is 10 g (males)/12 g (females).

iron-deficiency anemia: A form of anemia caused by insufficient levels of hemoglobin. Red blood cell count may be normal. Most commonly caused by inadequate intake or malabsorption of iron, or internal bleeding.

irrigation: The cleansing of a wound by flushing it with water, saline antiseptic, or other solution.

irritable bowel syndrome: Abnormal muscle contractions of the bowel causing abdominal pain and irregular bowel movements (diarrhea or constipation). There appears to be no physiological cause and there is no deterioration of general health. Often occurs due to stress or anxiety.

ischemia: Reduced oxygen supply to a tissue commonly due to constriction of blood vessels or edema.

isokinetic: A type of resistance exercise characterized by accommodating resistance throughout the full range of motion at a preset velocity (ie, the velocity remains constant while resistance varies according to the force output of the individual).

isometric: Literally means "same length" and refers to the length of the muscle. Isometric resistance exercise is characterized by a development of tension in a muscle without movement of related joints. Often used during periods of immobility to reduce atrophy.

isotonic: Literally means "same tension," however, in biomechanics it refers to resistance exercise in which concentric and eccentric exercises are performed against a constant weight.

itis: Suffix meaning "inflammation of."

J

Jackson's compression test: Special test of the cervical spine for nerve root compression. *See* Special Tests—Spine (Appendix 17).

JAT: Abbreviation for *Journal of Athletic Training*, the official journal of the National Athletic Trainers' Association.

jaundice: A condition characterized by a yellowing of the skin and whites of the eyes; excessive excretion of bilirubin by the liver, a common sign of liver disease.

Jerk Test of Hughston: A special test of the knee for the presence of ACL injury similar to the pivot shift test. The examiner applies a medial rotation force to the lower leg with the knee flexed to 90 degrees. Between 20 to 30 degrees the tibia shifts anteriorly and is reduced at full extension.

Jersey finger: A rupture of the flexor digitorum profundus tendon at the insertion. Characterized by an inability to flex the distal phalanx. Called Jersey finger due to the common mechanism of an athlete's finger getting caught in an opposing player's jersey.

Jobe relocation test: A special test for shoulder instability. *See* Special Tests—Shoulder (Appendix 17).

jock itch: *See* tinea cruris.

joint capsule: The fibrous tissue surrounding and providing stability to a joint.

joint mobilization: A manual therapy used to improve the accessory motions of sliding, spinning, and rolling.

joint play: The accessory movement that is necessary for physiological motion to occur; the amount of sliding, spinning, and rolling motion available in a joint.

joint position sense: The ability to detect actively or passively placed joint positions; a measure of proprioception.

Jones fracture: A transverse stress fracture of the fifth metatarsal.

JOSPT: Abbreviation for *Journal of Orthopedic and Sports Physical Therapy.*

joule: The international unit of work, energy; equal to the amount of work needed to move 1 Newton a distance of 1 meter or the work needed for 1 ampere to flow through the resistance of 1 ohm.

JRC-AT (Joint Review Committee on Educational Programs in Athletic Training): The professional review committee of the Commission on Accreditation of Allied Health Education Programs for athletic training.

JSR: Abbreviation for *Journal of Sport Rehabilitation.*

jumper's knee: The common term for tendinitis of the patella tendon.

Karnofsky scale: A rating used to determine a person's usual activities; used to evaluate progress.

Kehr's sign: Referred pain to the left shoulder from diaphragm or spleen injury or disease.

keloid: A firm, nodular scar formation with irregular bands of collagen that forms as a result of abnormal healing following an incision or burn.

Kendall test: A special test for rectus femoris tightness. *See* Special Tests—Hip (Appendix 17).

keratin: A scleroprotein found in nails and hair.

keratitis: Inflammation of the cornea.

keratosis: One of a number of abnormal, warty, pigmented growths on the skin, generally benign, however actinic keratosis may develop into squamous cell carcinoma if untreated.

Kernig sign: Special test of the spine for nerve root compression or irritation of the dura mater. *See* Special Tests—Spine (Appendix 17).

ketoacidosis (ketosis): Enhanced production of ketones sometimes occurring as a complication of diabetes mellitus.

kicker's knee: *See* patella tendonitis; also known as jumper's knee.

kidney stone: A hard, pebble-like mass commonly composed of calcium oxylate; also referred to as calculus; can be present in the kidney, ureter, or bladder causing severe pain (renal colic); in some cases must be removed surgically.

kilo: The SI unit for 1000.

kilocalorie (Kcal): A unit of measure for energy; equal to a nutritional calorie.

kinanesthesia: Inability to sense joint motions or positions.

kinematics: The study of the time and space factors related to motion.

kinesiology: The study of human movement.

kinesthesia: A sense of motion, velocity, and acceleration; kinesthesia is measured by "threshold to detection of passive movement."

kinesthetic awareness: The "sense" of body position or awareness, without which we would be unable to function with eyes closed.

kinetics: The study of the forces that cause motion.

Kleiger's test: A special test of the ankle ligaments. *See* Special Tests—Foot/Ankle (Appendix 17).

Klumpke palsy: A birth defect in which there is a lesion to the lower trunk of the brachial plexus or the nerve roots from C8-T1, causing weakness or paralysis of all ulnar innervated muscles as well as some of the distal median and radial innervated muscles.

kyphosis: The posterior curvature of the thoracic spine; increased kyphosis is often associated with a forward head posture and the cause of chronic neck and shoulder pain.

L

labyrinthitis: Inflammation of the labyrinth (inner ear) responsible for balance; can cause vertigo.

laceration: A torn or ragged open wound caused by blunt trauma.

Lachman's test: A special test of the knee for anterior cruciate injury. *See* Special Tests—Knee (Appendix 17).

lacrimation: An excess secretion of tears.

lactic acid: A byproduct of glucose metabolism in the absence of sufficient oxygen.

lactose: The disaccharide found in dairy milk.

lactose intolerance: A condition marked by the inability to break down and absorb the sugar lactose, causing cramping and diarrhea.

lamina: The posterior arch of vertebrae that connects the spinous process to the pedicle.

laminectomy: The surgical removal of the lamina of the spine, usually to gain access to a ruptured disc.

laparoscope: An instrument used to examine the abdominal cavity.

large intestine: The distal end of the alimentary canal between the small intestine and the anus consisting of the cecum, vermiform appendix, and colon.

Larsen-Johansson disease: Similar to Osgood-Schlatter disease, it is an apophysitis at the inferior pole of the patella.

laryngectomy: The surgical removal of all or part of the larynx, usually as a treatment for cancer.

laryngitis: Inflammation of the larynx causing one to lose his or her voice.

larynx: The organ between the pharynx and trachea that produces sound.

Lasegues test: Special test of the lumbar spine for nerve root compression. *See* Special Tests—Spine (Appendix 17).

laser (light amplification by stimulated emission of radiation): A form of treatment for surgery, cauterization, and treatment of skin wounds.

lateral: Toward the side of the body.

lateral epicondylitis: Inflammation of the lateral (extensor) epicondyle of the elbow. Common causes include repeated motion such as the force of deceleration during follow-through after hitting a backhand stroke in tennis (called tennis elbow).

lateral flexion: A flexion movement of the trunk or neck toward one side.

lateral longitudinal arch: The long arch along the lateral plantar surface of the foot created by the calcaneus, cuboid, third cuneiform, and the fourth and fifth metatarsals and supported by the long plantar ligament, the plantar calcaneocuboid ligament, the extensor digitorum tendons, and the interosseous muscles of the fifth toe.

lateral rotation: A rotation movement so as to turn the anterior aspect of the segment toward the outside or laterally; external rotation; outward rotation.

lateral spinothalmic tract: The tract or path of the spinal cord where Ad and C neurons synapse and send noxious stimuli to the brain.

Law of Grothus and Draper: Energy that is not absorbed will be transmitted to deeper tissues.

laxative: A pharmacological agent used to treat constipation or to clear the intestines prior to diagnostic procedures.

laxity: The state of being loose; the amount of joint play or joint movement.

LDL: *See* low-density lipoprotein.

left rotation: A rotation of the trunk or neck toward the left.

Legg-Calvé-Perthes disease: Coxa plana, or osteochondritis deformans juvenilis; avascular necrosis of the proximal femoral epiphysis occurring in boys 3 to 12 years of age.

Legionnaire's disease: A respiratory infection often leading to pneumonia that can be contracted through air-conditioning or water; named after the nationally publicized breakout at an American Legion convention in 1976.

leg length discrepancy: A measurable difference in bilateral leg length. Commonly measured as true leg length or real leg length. *See also* functional leg length and apparent leg length.

lesion: Any wound or injury; pathologic changes in a tissue.

leukemia: A proliferation of abnormal leukocytes affecting the production of normal white blood cells, red blood cells, and platelets; there are several varieties of leukemia.

leukocytes: White blood cells.

leukoplakia: Potentially cancerous white patches that develop in the mouth, vagina, or on the penis.

lever arm: *See* force arm.

lichen planus: Flat-topped, shiny eruptions found on male genitalia, flexor surfaces of the skin, and in the mouth that resolve spontaneously, sometimes months or years after their first appearance.

ligament: A tough, fibrous connective tissue that joins two or more bones at a joint.

Likert scale: A scale used to measure an individual's level of agreement or disagreement with a statement using a 3- or 5-point scale. Example: strongly disagree, disagree, neutral, agree, strongly agree.

linea alba: The median longitudinal tendinous line along the abdomen from the xiphoid to the pubic symphysis separating the two rectus abdominis muscles.

lipidosis: An abnormality of lipid metabolism that is hereditary in which fats are not properly broken down and thus there is an accumulation of lipids.

lipids: A group of fats that are stored in the body and used later for energy; they are important due to their association with vitamins and essential fatty acids.

lipoma: A benign fatty tumor.

lipoproteins: Important for the transport of lipids; one of many proteins that combine with lipids found in blood plasma and lymph.

liposarcoma: A malignant tumor of fatty tissue.

liposuction: A surgical procedure in which fat is removed by suction.

lipotropin: A substance in the anterior pituitary gland that stimulates the transport of stored fat to the bloodstream.

Lisfranc joint: The tarsometatarsal joints; articulation of the five metatarsal bases with the tarsal bones.

Lisfranc's fracture: A fracture and or displacement of one or more tarsometatarsal joints.

Lisinopril: An ACE inhibitor used to treat hypertension, heart failure, and acute myocardial infarction. Examples include Zestril (Zeneca Pharmaceuticals, Lincoln University, Pa) and Prinivil (Merck & Co, Inc, Whitehouse Station, NJ).

little league elbow: *See* medial epicondylitis.

liver: Large gland found in the upper right quadrant responsible for many vital functions such as synthesizing bile; metabolizing carbohydrates, proteins, and fats; controlling blood sugar by converting glucose to glycogen; and removing excess amino acids.

load-shift test: A special test of the shoulder in which the humeral head is gently pushed into the glenoid fossa and anterior and posterior translation is applied.

LOC: Abbreviation for loss of consciousness.

local anesthesia: A method of preventing pain by injecting a drug into or around a nerve, thereby reducing the loss of sensation in the area supplied by that nerve.

locomotor system: All of the components of the body segments responsible for moving the body as a whole.

long axis distraction: Distraction (traction) applied along the length of the bone.

longitudinal arch: The medial arch of the foot. *See* arch.

longitudinal axis: An imaginary line along the length of a body.

long thoracic nerve: The nerve supplying the serratus anterior, it arises from C5-7; injury to the long thoracic nerve results in characteristic "winging scapula" due to the inability to stabilize the scapula with the serratus anterior.

loose (open) packed position: A joint position when the joint surfaces are in a position of least congruency and at least part of the capsule is lax. In this position, the joint will exhibit the most laxity; *See* Appendix 16.

lordosis: The anterior curve of the lumbar spine.

Lou Gehrig's disease: *See* amyotrophic lateral sclerosis.

low dye technique: A taping procedure for the longitudinal arch.

low-density lipoprotein (LDL): The "bad" cholesterol; a lipoprotein that carries cholesterol in the blood; high levels of LDL are associated with heart disease and atherosclerosis.

lower motor neuron lesion (LMNL): A spinal cord lesion resulting in hyporeflexia, decrease in tone, or complete paralysis. Neuropraxia, axonotmesis, and neurotmesis are examples of LMNLs.

lower quarter screen: A quick check of the lower extremities to assist in localizing injury and to rule out gross neurological deficits. Includes thoracic and lumbar motions; isometric contraction of upper legs; movement of hip, knee, ankle, and foot. Sensory and reflex assessment. Heel and toe walking.

low-voltage current: Electrical stimulation using currents less than 150 volts.

Ludington's test: A special test of the shoulder to assess the integrity of the biceps tendon. A positive test indicates complete rupture of the biceps tendon. *See* Special Tests-Shoulder (Appendix 17).

lumbago: A term describing lower back pain.

lumbar plexus: A network of nerves made up of nerve roots L1-L4 that blend and divide to form a network.

lumbar spine: The last five vertebrae proximal to the sacrum.

lumbo-sacral plexus: The combination of the lumbar (L1-4) and sacral (L4-5, S1-4) plexes.

lupus: *See* systemic lupus erythematosus.

lupus erythematosus: An autoimmune disease characterized by chronic inflammation of connective tissue; can cause arthritis and progressive kidney damage.

luxation: Dislocation.

Lyme disease: A debilitating disease caused by the bacteria transmitted from a tick; signs and symptoms initially include flu-like symptoms followed by a characteristic "bulls-eye" lesion and rash, general malaise, and fatigue. If progression is not stopped, neurological changes including peripheral neuropathy, insomnia, and memory loss will occur. The end stages are characterized by symptoms similar to rheumatoid arthritis. Named for the location where it was first discovered, Lyme, Conn.

lymph: The clear, yellowish fluid in the lymphatic system that contains lymphocytes, otherwise similar to plasma with fewer proteins; contains white blood cells and antibodies that help fight against the spread of infection playing an important role in the immune system.

lymphadenitis: Inflammation of the lymph glands.

lymphadenopathy: The abnormal enlargement of a lymph node.

lymphatic system: The system made up of lymphatic vessels responsible for draining lymphatic fluid back into the blood.

lymph node: One of many small oval glands located along the lymphatic vessels.

lymphoma: A malignant tumor found in lymphoid tissue.

maculae: A spot; a small colored area.

magnetic resonance imaging (MRI): A technique that uses magnetic fields and radio frequencies to produce precise, high quality, cross-sectional images of the body.

main effects: In research, when a difference greater than that which could be expected due to error occurs across all levels of one of the factors.

malacia: Abnormal softening of a tissue.

malaise: Illness, discomfort.

malignant: A condition that is resistant to treatment and is characterized by uncontrolled growth, such as with cancer.

malingering: The act of pretending to be ill or injured, in order to be released from work or to gain attention.

mallet finger: A rupture of the extensor tendon causing a flexion of the DIP.

mallet toe: Similar to hammer toe but affects the distal interphalangeal joint of the toe, commonly the second toe; caused by neuropathy.

mammography: Imaging techniques including radiographic, ultrasound, and MRI techniques used for the diagnosis of breast disease.

mammoplasty: Any type of breast surgery or reconstruction including reduction, enlargement, and reconstruction after a mastectomy.

mandible: The bone of the lower jaw.

manic-depressive disorder: Bipolar disorder; a mental disorder in which the individual suffers from a shift between the two extremes of very high emotional "highs" and very low emotional "lows."

manipulation: A small amplitude, high force, passive therapy at the end range of motion for the purpose of restoring motion or improving position.

Mann-Whitney U: A nonparametric test of significance.

manual muscle testing (MMT): A form of resistive range of motion in which the examiner attempts to isolate individual muscles. *See* Appendix 6.

manual therapy: Therapeutic modalities that involve a "hands-on" approach. Joint mobilization and muscle energy are examples of manual therapy techniques.

manual traction: A manual therapy in which distractive (traction) forces are applied along the length of a bone or along joint segments. Commonly used to treat the spine by increasing joint space. This causes decreased pressure in the joint and stretching of the muscles, ligaments, and joint capsules.

march fracture: A stress fracture of a metatarsal; was commonly found in soldiers caused by prolonged marching.

Marfan syndrome: A rare genetic connective tissue disorder. A severe complication of aortic dilation and weakness, may cause an aneurysm to develop. Mitral valve prolapse is associated with this syndrome. Patient should be referred to physician and monitored very closely. Signs include abnormally long bones, concave chest, pes planus, and generalized joint hypermobility.

mass: The amount of matter; a measure of inertia.

mast cell: A large connective tissue cell containing heparin, histamine, and serotonin, important in the inflammatory process.

mastectomy: Surgical removal of all or part of the breast; *See also* modified radical mastectomy and radical mastectomy.

mastitis: Inflammation of the breast.

maxilla: A bilateral bone that forms half of the upper jaw and face as well as the roof of the mouth.

maximal voluntary contraction (MVC): The maximal amount of force possible exerted against a static force.

maximum compression test: Special test of the cervical spine for nerve root compression. *See* Special Tests—Spine (Appendix 17).

McBurney's point: A line between the umbilicus and ilium approximately 1 to 2 inches above the ASIS.

McConnell taping: Taping procedures designed to realign body structures; the most common procedure is used to treat patellofemoral dysfunction.

McKenzie extension exercises: Back and trunk exercises that emphasize extension with the intent of relieving pressure on the posterior wall of the disk.

McMurray's test: A special test of the knee to assess the presence of a meniscal tear. *See* Special Tests—Knee (Appendix 17).

mean: A statistical measure; the arithmetic average.

measles: A viral illness affecting primarily children, causing a characteristic rash and a fever; most Americans are inoculated against measles, mumps, and rubella (German measles).

mechanical advantage (MA): A situation in which a muscle is placed in a position such that it has an advantage due to the biomechanical arrangement. Such factors that affect mechanical advantage include muscle length, length of lever arm, and length of moment arm relative to the moment arm of the resistive force.

mechanical efficiency: The positioning of a limb or the body in such a way as to use the least energy in performing a given motion or to place the organ/tissue in a position of maximum advantage.

mechanical traction: A mechanical therapy in which a device is used to apply traction (distraction) forces between joints.

mechanoreceptor: A neuroreceptor that responds to mechanical stimuli such as touch, pressure, and tension.

medial: Toward the middle.

medial epicondylitis: Inflammation of the medial (flexor) epicondyle of the elbow. Often caused by the repeated forceful contractions during a flexion motion and/or flexion/pronation motion such as that during a pitch (little league elbow).

medial longitudinal arch: The long arch along the medial plantar surface of the foot from the calcaneus to the 1st to 3rd metatarsals including the talus, navicular, and three cuneiforms. The arch is supported by the plantar calcaneonavicular and deltoid ligaments, as well as the tendons of the tibialis posterior, tibialis anterior, and peroneus longus, and the interosseous muscles of the foot and plantar aponeurosis.

medial rotation: A rotation movement so as to turn the anterior aspect of the segment toward the inside or medially; internal rotation; inward rotation.

medial tibial stress syndrome: Also known as shin splints; an overuse syndrome of the muscles in the deep posterior compartment of the leg; often associated with pes planus and pronated feet.

median (Mdn): The middle score; the 50th percentile.

median nerve: One of the terminal branches of the brachial plexus arising from the nerve roots C5-T1. The median nerve crosses the wrist through the carpal tunnel and is affected by compression in carpal tunnel syndrome.

mediolateral: From medial to lateral.

MEDLINE: The online version of *Index Medicus*, it is a bibliographic database covering the fields of medicine, nursing, dentistry, veterinary medicine, the health care system, and the preclinical sciences containing over 4070 biomedical journals and over 11 million citations from 1960 to the present.

medulla: The bone marrow containing center of a longitudinal bone; the inner part of an organ, particularly the kidneys, adrenal gland, and lymph nodes; the distal end of the brainstem referring to the medulla oblongata.

melanin: The dark pigmentation of the skin, hair, and eyes.

melanoma: Malignant neoplasm that can form melanin most commonly in skin but frequently metastasizes to the lungs, lymph nodes, liver, and brain.

menarche: The onset of menstruation.

Meniere's disease: An inner ear disorder causing hearing loss, tinnitus, and dizziness.

meninges: The membranes of the spinal cord and brain (arachnoid, dura, and pia matters).

meningitis: Inflammation of the meninges; caused by bacterial or viral infection (bacterial is life-threatening while viral is often milder).

meniscectomy: The surgical removal or partial removal of the meniscus (usually of the knee).

meniscus: A crescent-shaped fibrocartilagenous in joints that helps to reduce friction; found in the knee and in the temporomandibular, sternoclavicular, and acromioclavicular joints.

menopause: The termination of menses.

menstruation: The cyclical (approximately monthly) occurrence in women that involves the endometrial shedding (the lining of the uterus).

mesomorph: A somatotype (ie, body type) commonly termed the "athletic build."

metabolic rate: How quickly the body uses energy.

metabolism: The chemical and physical processes that occur in the body and enable it to function and grow.

metabolite: Any product of metabolism.

metacarpals: The long bones of the hand just distal to the carpals and proximal to the phalanges.

metaphysis: The growing portion of a long bone found between the diaphysis and the epiphysis.

metastasis: The infiltration or spreading of cancer to another part of the body; as a noun it refers to a tumor that has occurred through this process.

metatarsal arch: Commonly referred to as the short lateral arch; formed by the heads of the metatarsals. However, there is disagreement as to whether this is an arch at all. Since the metatarsal heads are all weight-bearing, some believe there is no arch present.

metatarsals: The long bones of the foot just distal to the tarsals and proximal to the phalanges.

microbe: *See* microorganism.

microbiology: The study of microorganisms.

microcurrent electrical nerve stimulator (MENS): A type of electrical stimulator that delivers electrical current less than 1000 mA. Efficacy of MENS is inconclusive.

microorganism: Any microscopic, single-celled organism.

microsurgery: Surgery performed with the use of a microscope.

microwave diathermy: A deep heating modality from the electromagnetic spectrum that uses high frequency electromagnetic energy. Microwave diathermy has wavelengths ranging from 12 to 70 cm and operates at a frequency of approximately 430 to 2450 MHz.

mid stance: The mid point of the weightbearing phase of the walking cycle between heel strike and toe off.

migraine: A severe, often unilateral headache, usually accompanied by photophobia, phonophobia, nausea, vomiting, and dizziness.

mild brain injury (MBI): Concussion; brief loss of consciousness or a dazed feeling that can lead to post-concussion syndrome.

milliamp: Milliampere; one-thousandth of 1 ampere; unit of measure for electrical current.

mineral: An inorganic substance that serves as an important part of a healthy diet including potassium, calcium, sodium, phosphorus, and magnesium.

miotic: Drug-induced pupil constriction.

mitosis: The reproductive process of cell division.

mitral stenosis: A narrowing of the mitral valve causing the left atrium to work harder; an audible snap during diastole followed by a murmur can be heard during auscultation.

mitral valve: The valve in the heart that allows blood to flow from the left atrium to ventricle and prevents backflow.

mitral valve prolapse: A deformation of the mitral valve in the heart causing "a leak;" an audible murmur, chest pain, and abnormal heart rhythm are common.

MMR: Vaccination against measles, mumps, and rubella.

mobilization: The process of making a joint move more freely.

modality: A therapeutic agent used to reduce pain, swelling, and muscle spasm for the distinct purpose of promoting function.

mode: An approach to a treatment; in statistics, the score in a distribution that occurs most frequently.

modified radical mastectomy: A treatment for breast cancer similar to a radical mastectomy except the modified mastectomy leaves the pectoral muscles intact.

modified Romberg: A modification of the original Romberg test in which the patient is asked to stand on the limb of interest and maintain balance for a period of time (usually 20 to 30 seconds). This test is often performed with eyes closed in the case of assessing neuromuscular control following lower extremity injury.

modulation: In therapeutic modalities, the intentional alteration of one or more parameters in order to reduce the effect of accommodation.

mole: Nevus; a brown spot on the skin.

molecule: The smallest quantity of a substance that still retains its chemical properties.

molluscum contagiosum: An infectious disease characterized by dimpled papules. Caused by a pox virus and spread by human contact. May disappear spontaneously or surgical excision is required.

moment arm: *See* force arm.

mononucleosis: An acute infection caused by the Epstein-Barr virus in which there are large numbers of mononuclear leukocytes; symptoms include lethargy, fever, sore throat, and inflamed lymph nodes; the spleen can become enlarged with mononucleosis and persist up to 6 months.

monophasic current: An electrical current that does not cross the iso-electric line (ie, does not change polarity); has only one phase.

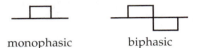

monophasic   biphasic

morbidity: Characteristic of illness or disease; the ratio of sick to healthy individuals in a given area.

morning sickness: A common occurrence of nausea and vomiting experienced early in a pregnancy.

mortality: A fatality; the state of being mortal; the death rate within a given population.

Morton's neuroma: A benign tumor on the common plantar nerve between the second and third or third and fourth metatarsal heads.

motive force: A force that causes motion. When lifting a weight against gravity, the muscles provide the motive force while gravity provides a resistive force. When lowering a weight with gravity, gravity provides the motive force, while the muscles provide a resistive force.

motor control: The neurophysiological factors that affect human movement, specifically the interaction between the brain and musculoskeletal system during performance of isolated tasks.

motor development: The study of changes in motor behavior over the entire life span.

motor learning: The study of the processes involved in learning and mastering new skills.

motor neuron: An efferent nerve cell that sends signals from the central nervous system to a muscle

motor unit: An alpha motor neuron, its axon, and all the muscle fibers attached to it.

MS: *See* multiple sclerosis.

mucous membrane: Mucosa; the moist lining of many tubular structures consisting of an epithelial layer that contains secreting glands and deeper layers of connective tissue.

mucus: A clear secretion produced by mucous membranes that forms a protective barrier that lubricates and carries enzymes.

multiarticulate: Referring to the crossing of multiple joints. For example, the biceps brachii is considered multiarticulate due to the fact that it crosses and performs a function at the shoulder joint (shoulder flexion), radioulnar joint (supination), and ulnohumeral joint (elbow flexion).

multiple regression: A regression analysis on one dependent variable and multiple independent variables.

multiple sclerosis (MS): A demyelinating disease that affects the central nervous system. Patients suffer cycles of relapse followed by remission.

mumps: A common viral infection primarily affecting children that causes fever, nausea, vomiting, and characteristic inflammation of salivary glands; immunity is usually developed through a childhood infection.

murmur: A characteristic abnormal blood flow sound heard during auscultation.

Murphy's sign: A special test for lunate injury. *See* Special Tests—Hand/Wrist (Appendix 17).

muscle energy techniques: A treatment technique used to improve function by directing the concentrated muscular efforts of the patient at precise positions.

muscle relaxants: A pharmacologic agent used to reduce tension in the muscles.

muscle spindles: A stretch-sensitive receptor.

muscle strength: The maximum tension that can be produced by a muscle or muscle group.

muscle testing: *See* manual muscle testing.

muscle tone: A normal state of tension in a muscle that is controlled by reflex activity.

muscle wasting: Atrophy, the degeneration of a muscle.

muscular dystrophy (MD): An inherited disease in which there is marked muscle wasting. There are several variations of the disease; Duchenne's dystrophy is the most common, affecting primarily young boys.

muscular endurance: The ability of a muscle to contract repeatedly.

musculocutaneous nerve: One of the terminal branches of the brachial plexus arising from the nerve roots C5-C7. The musculocutaneous nerve innervates the biceps brachii and the coracobrachialis muscles.

MVC: *See* maximal voluntary contraction.

myalgia: Muscular pain.

myasthenia gravis: A disease in which there is marked weakness and fatigability of the muscles. Drooping of the upper eyelid is a common sign. Adolescent and young adult females are most often affected.

mycosis: A fungal disease.

myelin sheath: The outer covering, made of fat and protein, that surrounds and protects some nerves and improves conduction velocity.

myelitis: Inflammatory disease of the spinal cord common in multiple sclerosis but can occur in its absence; symptoms include headache, fever, muscle stiffness, pain, weakness, and eventually complete paralysis below the level of the disease; also refers to inflammation of the bone marrow (osteomyelitis).

myelocele: A neural tube defect; a severe form of spina bifida in which there is a protrusion of the meninges surrounding the spinal cord, and the spinal cord and nerves roots are exposed.

myelogram: A radiography of the spine following injection of contrast medium. Used rarely since the advent of CT scan and MRI.

myeloma: A tumor originating in blood cells in the bone marrow.

myelomalacia: A softening of the spinal cord.

myelomeningocele: Spina bifida including protusions of portions of the spinal cord and surrounding membranes.

myelosclerosis: Myelofibrosis; sclerosis of the bone marrow affecting the production of blood and its components.

myocardial infarction (MI): Commonly called a heart attack; a sudden insufficiency of blood and oxygen to an area of the heart causing tissue necrosis.

myocarditis: Inflammation of the heart muscle; can be caused by drugs, a virus, or radiation.

myocardium: Heart muscle.

myofascial release (MFR): A manual therapy in which deep friction massage is used to improve the mobility of fascial and muscular tissues.

myopathy: A muscle disease, usually one that results in muscle atrophy.

myopia: A condition commonly known as near-sightedness; it is caused by visual images coming into focus in front of the retina, resulting in blurred vision especially of objects at a distance.

myositis: Inflammation of a muscle or muscles causing pain and loss of strength.

myositis ossificans: Inflammation in a muscle leading to ossification. A common complication to severe thigh contusions.

myotome: The group of muscles innervated by a nerve root.

N

Naproxen: Naprosyn; a nonsteroidal anti-inflammatory medication.

narcolepsy: A disorder that causes uncontrollable episodes of falling asleep during the day.

narcosis: A drug-induced stupor or sleepiness.

narcotic: A substance with addictive properties known for its ability to dull the senses. A narcotic analgesic, for example, blocks the transmission of pain.

nares: Openings in the nose.

nasal septum: The cartilage/bone central divider of the nasal passage.

nasopharynx: The passageway from the nasal passage to the back of the throat.

nates: The buttocks.

natural immunity: Immunity to a disease by virtue of belonging to a particular race or species or an acquired immunity due to exposure to infection.

nausea: A sick feeling characterized by the need to vomit.

necrosis: Tissue death.

Neer's impingement test: A special test of the shoulder used to assess the presence of impingement. *See* Special Tests—Shoulder (Appendix 17).

neoplasm: An abnormal growth; tumor.

nephrectomy: The surgical removal of a kidney.

nephritis: Inflammation of the kidney.

nephroblastoma: "Wilm's tumor"; a fast-growing tumor of the kidneys affecting primarily children under 4 years old and rarely seen in children over the age of 18.

nephrolithotomy: Surgical removal of a kidney stone.

nephrology: The study of kidney disease.

nephron: The active filtering unit of the kidneys.

nephrosclerosis: A "hardening of the arteries" of the kidneys associated with hypertension.

nephrostomy: The surgical placement of a catheter directly into the kidney through the skin.

nerve: A bundle of fibers that transmit electrical impulses to and from the brain body tissues. Afferent nerves convey sensory information from the periphery to the brain while efferent nerves convey impulses from the brain to the periphery, especially muscles to provide motor function.

nerve block: A procedure used to reduce pain by injecting a local anesthetic into or around a nerve causing local analgesia.

nerve cell: A neuron; a specialized cell (composed of a cell body or soma, an axon, and one or more dendrites) that transmits electrical impulses from one area of the body to another.

nerve compression: Injury to a nerve induced by pressure, causing pain, weakness, or paresthesia.

neuralgia: A severe, sharp, or deep pain that follows a nerve distribution.

neurapraxia: Commonly referred to as a burner, stinger, or pinched nerve; a transient nerve compression or stretch causing pain, paresthesia, and weakness.

neuritis: Inflammation of a nerve, characterized by pain, numbness, or paresthesia.

neurogenic: Caused by or related to nerve injury.

neurogenic pain: Pain caused by injury to or illness of the nervous system.

neuroma: A benign tumorous growth from the fibrous covering of a peripheral nerve.

neuromuscular: Pertaining to the interaction and coordination of the nervous and muscular systems.

neuromuscular control: The efferent responses to the sensory information provided by kinesthesia and proprioception.

neuromuscular electrical stimulator (NMES): A type of electrical modality designed specifically to produce muscular contraction used to reeducate, strengthen, or maintain strength during periods of immobility, and to reduce spasticity.

neuron: Another term for a nerve cell; a specialized cell of the nervous system that carries information to and from the central nervous system, composed of a cell body (soma), an axon, and one or more dendrites.

neurons: Nerve cell; unit of the nervous system consisting of the cell body, the axon, and one or more dendrites.

neuropathy: Disease or injury to peripheral nerves causing pain, numbness, and weakness.

neuropraxia: A lower motor neuron lesion.

neurosis: A psychological disorder in which insight is retained. Examples include mild depression, obsessive-compulsive disorder, and phobias.

neurotmesis: A lower motor neuron lesion.

neurotoxin: A poisonous or harmful chemical that attacks and damages nerve cells.

neurotransmitter: A chemical mediator that aids in the transmission of electrical impulses across the synapse. Examples include acetylcholine, norepinephrine, dopamine, and serotonin.

neurotrophic: Relating to the growth and nutrition of nervous tissue.

neutrophil: A white blood cell that ingests bacteria and thus helps fight infection; there are 2.0 to 7.5 x 109 neutrophils per liter of blood.

Niacin: Nicotinic acid; also known as vitamin B_3; dietary sources include meat, peanut butter, and enriched cereals; the RDA for an adult is 18 mg/day; deficiencies lead to pellagra.

Noble's compression test: A special test of the knee used to assess IT band friction syndrome. *See* Special Tests—Knee (Appendix 17).

nociceptors: Afferent nerves responsible for sensing pain.

node: A small, rounded tissue mass.

node of Ranvier: The break or gap that occurs at the end of the Schwan cell in myelinated nerves.

nodule: A small lump caused by a group of cells or swelling of tissue that is usually abnormal.

nominal data: Data values that represent categories in which no intrinsic order exists. A type of nonparametric measure in which observations are classified according to a characteristic such as male or female, injured or not injured.

noninsulin-dependent diabetes: Also known as type II diabetes; a type of diabetes mellitus that occurs mainly in overweight adults over age 40 that can be treated with changes to the diet and the use of other drugs to increase natural production of insulin.

noninvasive: A medical procedure that does not involve penetration of the body; also used to refer to benign tumors that have remained localized.

nonnarcotic analgesic: A pharmacological agent that inhibits the release of neurotransmitters responsible for stimulating pain-sensing nerves and thus causes a relief of pain.

nonsteroidal anti-inflammatory drugs (NSAIDs): One of the many anti-inflammatory drugs that is not from the steroid family; used to reduce inflammation and pain. Examples include aspirin (acetylsalicylic acid), ibuprofen, naproxen sodium, piroxicam, and sulindac.

norepinephrine: A hormone secreted by the medulla responsible for the regulation of blood pressure.

normal force: The force directed perpendicular to a surface.

nosebleed: *See* epitaxis.

notch: An indentation in a bone.

nucleic acids: DNA or RNA present in the nucleus responsible for heredity.

nucleus: The DNA- and RNA-containing center of a cell.

nutrient: A substance required by the body to maintain its health, including carbohydrates, fats, proteins, minerals, and vitamins.

nystagmus: Involuntary lateral movement of the eyes.

Ober's test: A special test of the hip used to assess tensor fascia tightness. *See* Special Tests—Hip (Appendix 17).

obesity: A condition in which a person is more than 20% above the normal body weight for his or her age, height, and gender.

objective measure: A measurement technique that does not allow feelings or opinions (bias) of the investigator to affect the outcome; a test with precise scoring.

O'Brien test: A special test of the shoulder used to test for a SLAP lesion. *See* Special Tests—Shoulder (Appendix 17).

OBS: Abbreviation for "organic brain syndrome" or "observation."

obsessive-compulsive disorder: A tendency to perform repetitive behaviors to relieve anxiety, such as constantly washing the hands for fear of germs or repeatedly checking to see if the oven has been turned off or the door is locked; an unnatural concern that things are in order or in their exact place.

obturator nerve: The peripheral nerve from the lumbosacral plexus that innervates the hip adductors.

occlusion: To close; the state of being closed.

ocular: Of or pertaining to the eyes.

oculomotor nerve: Cranial nerve III responsible for voluntary motor control of the eyes. *See* Appendix 8.

ohm: A measure of the resistance to current flow.

olfactory nerve: Cranial nerve I responsible for the sense of smell. *See* Appendix 8.

oligomenorrhea: Infrequent menstruation.

one-tail (directional) test: A test for significance in which direction is predicted. It uses only one tail of the normal curve.

oocyte: A not quite fully developed egg cell; also called ovocyte. *See* primary oocyte and secondary oocyte.

oophorectomy: The surgical removal of an ovary.

open (kinetic) chain: An exercise in which the distal end is free to move. Example: knee extension or hamstring curls.

open (loose) packed position: A joint position when the bone ends in a position of least congruency. In this position, the joint will exhibit the most laxity. *See* Appendix 16.

ophthalmia: Inflammation of the eye, usually involving deeper structures; a severe conjunctivitis.

ophthalmic nerve: A small branch of the trigeminal nerve.

ophthalmologist: A physician specializing in ophthalmology.

ophthalmology: A medical specialty concerned with diseases and injuries of the eye.

ophthalmoscope: A medical instrument used to examine the interior aspect of the eye.

Oppenheim's reflex: A reflex test in which the examiner runs a fingernail along the anterior tibia. A positive test is indicated by a positive Babinski's sign. *See also* Babinski's reflex/sign.

opposition: Movement of the thumb toward the palm of the hand.

optic: Relating to the eye.

optician: A specialist who makes and fits ophthalmic lenses.

optic nerve: Cranial nerve II responsible for controlling the visual acuity. *See* Appendix 8.

optic neuritis: Inflammation of the optic nerve; often results in some vision loss.

ordinal data: Data values that represent categories that include some intrinsic order. For example: strongly disagree, disagree, neutral, agree, strongly agree.

origin: A place of muscular attachment to a bone. The muscular attachment on the fixed segment or the attachment nearest the midline of the trunk.

oropharynx: The middle portion of the pharynx between the palate and the upper epiglottis.

orthotic: Orthosis; an external device used to correct or control biomechanics by limiting movement, providing support, increasing velocity or power, or generally enhancing function.

os: Bone; mouth-like.

Osgood-Schlatter disease/syndrome: An apophysitis of the tibial tubercle caused by excessive repeated strain and seen most often in adolescents.

osmosis: The process of the passage of substances through a semi permeable membrane from an area of lesser concentration to an area of higher concentration.

ossification: The formation or maintenance of bone.

osteitis: Inflammation of the bone.

osteitis deformans: Paget's disease; a progressive disorder of abnormal bone growth resulting in a thickening and softening of bones.

osteitis pubis: An overuse inflammatory process to the muscular attachment of several muscles that attach to the pubic symphysis.

osteoarthritis: A form of degenerative arthritis affecting joint cartilage and, subsequently, the underlying bone.

osteoblast: A cell responsible for bone formation.

osteochondritis dissecans: Degeneration within a joint in which there are small fragments of bone and cartilage in the joint causing pain, swelling, and loss of range of motion.

osteochondroma: A benign bone and cartilage tumor.

osteoclast: A cell responsible for breaking down unwanted bony tissue; a medical device used to correct bony deformity by fracturing the bone.

osteoma: A benign tumor of the bone.

osteomalacia: Softening of bones and loss of minerals due to vitamin D deficiency (also known as rickets in children).

osteomyelitis: Bacterial-induced inflammation affecting both bone and bone marrow.

osteonecrosis: Death of bone tissue.

osteophyte: A bony outgrowth near a joint, related to cartilage degeneration.

osteoporosis: A condition in which there is loss of bone tissue causing bones to become brittle and less dense, leading to fractures.

os trigonum: The posterior process of the talus that serves as a site of attachment for the posterior talofibular ligament; it sometimes becomes separated from the talus to form this small triangular bone.

otitis externa: Known as "swimmer's ear"; inflammation of the outer ear due to an infection.

otitis media: Inflammation of the middle ear often caused by nose and throat infection.

otoscope: A medical instrument used to examine the ear.

outcome measure: A means of assessment by evaluating the success of the treatment or program.

outward rotation: A rotation movement so as to turn the anterior aspect of the segment toward the outside or laterally; lateral rotation; external rotation.

ovaries: Bilateral glands at the opening of the fallopian tubes of the uterus responsible for production of eggs and the hormones estrogen and progesterone.

overpressure: A technique of applying pressure to a joint at its end range of motion to assess the end feel. *See* End Feel (Appendix 15).

over-the-counter: Pertaining to a medication that can be purchased without a physician's prescription.

overuse syndrome: A chronic injury caused by repetitive stress. Examples of overuse syndromes include tendonitis, lateral epicondylitis (tennis elbow), medial tibial stress syndrome, medial epicondylitis (little league elbow), carpal tunnel syndrome, Osgood-Schlatter, and pronator teres syndrome.

ovulation: Release of an ovum, usually occurring around midcycle.

ovum: Egg cell.

pacemaker: A small electronic device surgically implanted to produce and maintain a normal heart rhythm.

Paget's disease: A metabolic bone disorder occurring in the middle-aged and elderly in which bone does not form properly, causing bone weakening, thickening, and deformity; osteitis deformans.

painful arc test: A special test of the shoulder in which the examiner notes the portion of the range of motion in which the patient exhibits pain.

pain scale: A scale used to assess the relative pain of an individual. One example, shown below, is the visual analog scale consisting of a 10-cm line with descriptors on either end. Another example is a numeric pain scale ranging from 1 (no pain) to 10 (worst pain imaginable).

visual analog scale

no pain   worst pain imaginable

palate: The roof of the mouth.

pallor: Pale skin, especially the face.

palpate: The act of using the hands or fingertips to discriminate tissue tension; to assess swelling, temperature, and to determine if point tenderness is present.

palpitation: An abnormally rapid and strong heartbeat.

palsy: Paralysis.

pancreas: A gland located behind the stomach in the upper left quadrant responsible for the production of enzymes that help to break down food and hormones; responsible for the regulation of glucose levels by the release of insulin and glucagons.

pancreatitis: Inflammation of the pancreas, often caused by alcoholism.

panic disorder: An emotional disorder characterized by anxiety attacks, often brought about by stress.

papilloma: A tumor, usually benign, found on skin and mucous membranes.

pap smear: A medical procedure in which epithelial cells are scraped from the cervix for examination to detect abnormal changes.

para: Beside, next to; abbreviation for "paraplegia."

paraffin bath: The use of melted paraffin wax as a thermo-therapeutic modality.

paralysis: Muscle weakness or an inability to contract a muscle or group of muscles including increased tone (spasticity) and decreased tone (flaccidity).

paramedical: Relating to the professions of individuals who have special training to provide various medical care but do not have a medical degree. Examples include nurses, physical therapists, athletic trainers, and emergency medical technicians.

paranoia: A psychosis characterized by unfounded suspicions of others.

paraplegia: Partial or complete loss of motor and sensory function of the legs.

parasite: An organism that inhabits and obtains its nutrients from another organism.

parasympathetic nervous system: The part of the autonomic nervous system that frequently opposes the sympathetic nervous system functioning mainly during relaxation.

parathyroidectomy: The surgical removal of a parathyroid gland.

parathyroid glands: Two pairs of small glands found in or near the thyroid that are stimulated to release parathyroid hormone by reductions of calcium in the blood.

parathyroid hormone: A hormone released by the parathyroid glands that controls the level of calcium in the blood.

parenteral: A substance administered by any route other than through the mouth.

paresis: Loss of muscle strength; partial paralysis.

paresthesia: Tingling sensation; "pins and needles," loss of normal sensation.

Parkinson's disease: A disease of the basal ganglia. Symptoms include tremor and rigidity beginning in one arm and eventually affecting all limbs; caused by a lack of the chemical mediator dopamine.

paronychia: Bacterial or fungal infection, most commonly staphylococci or streptococci, causing inflammation around the nail beds.

passive range or motion (PROM): Range of motion performed by the examiner in which the patient remains relaxed. PROM is used to assess inert tissue.

passive stretch: A stretch to improve range of motion in which no active muscular contraction takes place.

patella: Kneecap.

patella alta: An abnormally high position of the patella in its groove.

patella baja: An abnormally low position of the patella in its groove.

pathogen: The microorganism or bacteria that causes disease.

pathogenesis: The process of the development of a disease or disorder.

pathology: The study of disease processes in order to understand the cause.

Patrick's test: *See* FABRE.

PDR (*Physician's Desk Reference*): A reference text for prescription drugs, published annually.

peak flow measurement: A method used to determine the maximum velocity that air is exhaled from a patient's lungs; used to diagnose lung conditions or to determine the effectiveness of medications to treat the condition.

Pearson r: A statistical measure of the correlation between two sets of parametric data.

pediculosis: Commonly called lice, an infection of the scalp caused by parasite. Spreads through shared uses of hats, combs, brushes, etc. Common in school-aged children.

peer review: An assessment of a body of work by a colleague with equal status.

pellagra: Vitamin B_3 (niacin) deficiency causing dermatitis, diarrhea, and depression.

pelvic inflammatory disease (PID): The result of a bacterial infection; an inflammation of the reproductive organs in females; the use of tampons is linked to PID.

pelvic obliquity: A deviation between the spine and pelvis in the frontal plane genrealy caused by contractures.

pepsin: The enzyme that helps digest protein.

peptic ulcer: A break or erosion of the mucosa caused by abnormally high concentrations of pepsin and acid.

perceived exertion: A measure used to assess an individual's perception of his or her exertion. *See* rating of perceived exertion and Borg scale.

perceptual motor skill: An activity that relies on special orientation, ocular control, and perception of body position in relation to the environment.

percussion: A diagnostic technique that involves tapping the surface to determine density of an area.

percutaneous: Through the skin.

perforation: The creation of a hole in an organ or body tissue caused by disease or injury.

periaqueductal grey (PAG): A midbrain structure important in the central biasing pain control theory in which descending impulses are initiated that travel down the dorsal horn to inhibit synaptic transmission of pain.

pericarditis: Inflammation of the membrane that surrounds the heart, causing chest pain and fever.

periodontitis: Inflammation and/or degeneration of the dental periosteum often caused by chronic gingivitis or poor hygiene.

periosteum: The outer covering of bone.

periostitis: Inflammation of the periosteum.

peripheral nervous system: The nervous system outside of the central nervous system, including the cranial nerves, spinal nerves, and all of its roots.

peripheral vascular disease: Reduced blood flow to the extremities due to a narrowing of the blood vessels, leading to pain and tissue damage in which necrosis may ensue.

peristalsis: A wave-like movement characteristic of tube-like structures for the purpose of moving material within the tube. The muscles immediately behind a material contract, and the ones immediately in front of a material relax.

peritoneum: The serous membrane that lines the abdomen.

peritonitis: Inflammation of the peritoneum.

pernicious: Describes serious diseases that are likely to result in death if untreated.

peroneal: Relating to the lateral (fibular) aspect of the lower leg.

peroneal nerve, common: One of the branches from the sciatic nerve; wraps around the fibular head before further dividing into the deep and superficial peroneal nerves; deep—found in the anterior compartment, innervates the tibialis anterior, the extensor hallicus longus, extensor digitorum, and the peroneus tertius; superficial—found in the lateral compartment, innervates peroneus longus and brevis.

peroneus: One of the lateral muscles of the lower leg. The peroneus longus and brevis cross the ankle posterior to the lateral malleolus and thus are responsible for plantar flexion and eversion of the ankle. The peroneus tertius lies just anterior to the lateral malleolus as it crosses the ankle and is thus responsible for dorsiflexion and eversion. The peroneus longus and brevis are innervated by the surperficial peroneal nerve while the peroneus tertius is innervated by the deep peroneal nerve.

Perthes' disease: *See* Legg-Calvé-Perthes disease.

pes: Foot.

pes anserine: Literally "foot of a bird"; the insertion of the semitendinosis, sartorius, and gracilis to the anteromedial tibia.

pes cavus: Abnormally high arches.

pes planus: Flat feet.

petit mal: A type of seizure characterized by a brief loss of awareness with no loss of consciousness.

petrissage: A type of therapeutic massage involving a kneading type of motion.

pH: A measure of the concentration of hydrogen in a solution; a pH less than 7 indicates an acidic solution and above 7 indicates an alkaline solution.

phagocyte: A cell that plays an important role in the healing process by digesting debris, microorganisms, and other unwanted material.

phalanges: The small bones of the fingers and toes.

Phalen's test: A special test of the wrist and hand to assess carpal tunnel syndrome. *See* Special Tests— Hand/Wrist (Appendix 17).

phantom limb: A sensation after a limb has been amputated that the limb still exists.

pharmacology: The study of the properties and actions of drugs.

pharyngitis: Inflammation of the pharynx, accompanied by sore throat, swollen glands, fever, and earache.

pharynx: The throat; a hollow tube that acts as the food and air passageway from the mouth and nose to the esophagus and larynx.

phases: In therapeutic modalities, a portion of a wave, or pulse. A pulse consisting of one phase is termed *monophasic*; two phases, *biphasic*; and more than two phases is termed *polyphasic*.

phenylketonuria: A hereditary disorder in which the individual cannot convert the amino acid phenylalanine and therefore it must not be consumed.

phlebitis: Inflammation of a vein.

phlebothrombosis: A blood clot in a vein.

phlegm: Sputum.

phobia: An unfounded fear of an event or situation. Phobias can have a profound effect on one's life because of the strong desire to avoid these situations.

phonophoresis: The use of ultrasound to deliver medication to deeper tissues.

photophobia: Oversensitivity of the eyes to light.

photosensitivity: An abnormal sensitivity to sunlight that results in skin irritation and rash.

phototherapy: An intervention with some form of light.

physical activity: Defined by the NATA as athletic, recreational, or occupational activities that require physical skills and utilize strength, power, endurance, speed, flexibility, range of motion, or agility.

physically active: Defined by the NATA as individuals engaged in athletic, recreational, or occupational activities that require physical skills and utilize strength, power, endurance, speed, flexibility, range of motion, or agility.

physical therapy: The treatment of injuries or disorders using mechanical treatments, including exercise, massage, manual therapies, mobilization, or the application of therapeutic modalities.

physiological motion: The voluntary motions such as flexion, extension, abduction, adduction, etc. Physiological motions require accessory motions.

physiology: The study of the functioning of living organisms.

piezoelectric effect: The vibration of the crystal in an ultrasound head when electrical current passes through it.

pinched nerve: *See* neurapraxia.

pinch test: A special test of the wrist and hand to assess the median nerve or carpal tunnel syndrome. *See* Special Tests—Hand/Wrist (Appendix 17).

pinkeye: *See* conjunctivitis.

pinna: Cartilaginous portion of the external ear.

pinna hematoma: *See* auricular hematoma.

PIP: Abbreviation for proximal interphalangeal joint.

piriformis syndrome: The compression of the sciatic nerve from the piriformis muscle caused by inflammation or hypertrophy. In some individuals, the sciatic nerve pierces the piriformis muscle.

pitting edema: A thick viscous type of swelling associated with lymphedema that leaves an indentation (or "pit") when the skin is depressed during palpation.

pityriasis: Skin disease characterized by bran-like scales. Pityriasis alba is very common in children and adolescents and is characterized by pale macules on the face. Pityriasis rosea is a mild skin condition occurring in adults in which flat, scaly macules occur on the trunk and upper arms.

pivot shift test: A special test of the knee to assess the anterior cruciate ligament (ACL). *See* Special Tests—Knee (Appendix 17).

PKU: *See* phenylketonuria.

placebo: A sham treatment or chemically inactive substance given to a subject in a clinical trial. A placebo effect is the positive or negative response to the treatment due to the expectations of the treatment rather than the treatment itself.

planes of motion: *See* cardinal planes.

plantar fascia: A strong fibrous connective tissue on the plantar surface of the foot that runs from the medial tubercle of the calcaneus to the proximal metatarsal heads.

plantar wart: A wart on the sole of the foot, frequently painful and covered by callus.

plethysmography: A measurement technique for limb volume due to changes in blood pressure.

pleura: The membrane that surrounds both lungs.

pleurisy: Inflammation of the pleura. Also called *pleuritis*.

plexus: A network of nerves or blood vessels.

plica: A fold in the synovial tissue. A plica in the knee is a common site of pain.

plyometric: A type of exercise in which a quick stretch (or lengthening) is used just prior to the forceful contraction.

PMS: *See* premenstrual syndrome.

pneumonia: A bacterial or viral infection of the lungs classified by site and causative factors. There are more than 25 classifications. Common symptoms include fever, shortness of breath, and cough although not all patients exhibit these symptoms. Most common in the elderly and individuals with weakened systems.

pneumonitis: Inflammation of the lungs.

pneumothorax: A condition in which air enters the pleural cavity, causing chest pain and shortness of breath.

PNF: *See* proprioceptive neuromuscular facilitation.

point tenderness: The pain that is produced when an area is palpated.

poliomyelitis: Commonly referred to as polio; an infectious viral disease of the motor cells of the spinal cord.

pollex: The thumb.

polycystic kidney disease: Multiple cysts on the kidneys.

polycystic ovary syndrome: Multiple cysts on the ovaries.

polycythemia: Excessive hemoglobin concentration.

polydipsia: Excessive thirst.

polymyalgia rheumatica: A rare disease affecting older adults resulting in generalized pain and stiffness in the hips, thighs, shoulders, and neck.

polyneuritis: Inflammation of multiple nerves.

polyp: A tumor projecting from a mucous membrane that can become cancerous.

polyuria: Excessive production of urine, a common sign of diabetes mellitus and other diseases.

pons: A tissue "process" connecting two or more segments or parts. In the brain it connects the medulla to the cerebellum and contains the origins of the abducens, facial, trigeminal, and cochlear portion of the vestibulo-cochlear cranial nerve at its border.

post-concussion syndrome: Symptoms following a mild head injury that can include headaches, dizziness, mild mental impairment (difficulty concentrating), and fatigue lasting a few months to indefinitely.

posterior: Back, dorsal.

posterior draw (drawer) sign: A special test of the knee to assess the posterior cruciate ligament (PCL). *See* Special Tests—Knee (Appendix 17).

posteroanterior: From back to front.

post-traumatic amnesia: Loss of memory or state of confusion following traumatic brain injury caused by inflammation, disruption of blood flow, or disruption of brain, or neural tissue. Usually resolves within a few weeks but can last up to several months.

post-traumatic stress disorder (PTSD): A condition following a frightening or stressful life event in which the individual suffers from recurring dreams, difficulty sleeping, "flashbacks," and fear of recurrence of the event.

postural sway: A measure of balance, generally a measure of the time and distance excursion from one's center of balance.

posture: The attitude of the body; the position maintained by the body in standing or in sitting; the alignment and positioning of the body in relation to gravity, center of mass, and base of support; the position of the body or body part in relation to space and/or to other body parts. Functionally, the anticipation about, in response to, displacement of the body's center of mass.

Pott's fracture: A fracture of the distal fibula and medial malleolus of the tibia with an outward displacement of the foot.

power: The amount of work performed per unit of time. $p = (w \times d)/time$.

predictor: A variable used to predict behavior.

premenopausal: The period that accounts for the years leading up to menopause.

premenstrual syndrome: The physical and emotional symptoms that occur 7 to 14 days prior to menstruation or from ovulation to the onset of menstruation; symptoms include depression, irritability, abdominal pain, and fatigue.

presbyopia: Also known as far-sightedness; the degradation of near vision occurring naturally with age due to a loss of elasticity of the lens of the eyes, generally resulting in the need for reading glasses.

pressure: The ratio of force to the area where the force is applied.

pressure point (trigger point): A tender point that has a relationship to an area of pain.

primary oocyte: The ovum at the end of maturation but before the first division of meiosis.

primary survey: The initial assessment of an injured or ill individual that assesses immediate and life threatening conditions. Includes surveying the scene, determining level of consciousness, presence of breathing, pulse, bleeding, and observation for immediate life threatening conditions.

prime mover: A muscle primarily responsible for a given movement; example: the biceps brachii muscle is a prime mover for elbow flexion.

profile test: A special test for posterior cruciate ligament instability. Also called Sag test. *See* Special Tests—Knee (Appendix 17).

prognosis: An assessment of the probable outcome of the patient's disease.

progressive resistance exercise (PRE): Developed by Delorme, it is an exercise method consisting of the use of weights lifted through a range of motion against gravity. The amount of weight and the number of repetitions is progressively increased as follows: First set, 10 reps at 50% of 10 repetitions maximum (RM); second set, 10 reps at 75% of 10 RM; third set at 100% of 10 RM. The Oxford technique is the same except the percentages are performed in reverse order. *See also* DAPRE.

prolapse: Disc herniation of the nucleus pulposus through the annulus fibrosis.

pronation (of the arm): Internal rotation of the forearm so as to place the palm down.

pronation (of the foot): The act of turning downward; in the foot, pronation is dependent upon whether the motion is performed open or closed chain. During closed chain movement, pronation involves plantar flexion, eversion, and adduction. During open chain movement, pronation involves dorsiflexion, eversion, and abduction.

pronator teres syndrome: A compression of the median nerve by the pronator teres muscle.

prone: With the front or ventral surface down; lying face down.

prophylactic: Preventative measure.

proprioception: A sense or awareness of position.

proprioceptive neuromuscular facilitation (PNF): A method of using passive, active, and active-assisted range of motion to improve flexibility and neuromuscular strength. There are many techniques of PNF.

proprioceptor: A receptor that responds to changes in the body such as movement and position.

prostate gland: An accessory gland located under the bladder and vas deferens in men. It is responsible for the production of part of the semen. It can become enlarged in older men, impairing urination and subsequently causing damage to the kidneys.

prosthesis: A device used to improve function and/or to replace a missing or impaired organ or body part.

proteinemia: Excess protein in the blood.

proteinuria: Protein in the urine.

protraction: Abduction of the scapula.

protusion: The least severe disc herniation in which the nucleus pulposus does not actually exit through the annulus fibrosis, rather a "bulge" puts pressure on the nerve root.

proximal: A term of description denoting a segment or body part that is nearer the central point (or core); closer to the point of origin.

pruritus: Itching.

psoriasis: A chronic skin disorder characterized by itchy, scaly, red patches most commonly found on the elbows, knees, forearms, legs, and scalp.

psoriatic arthritis: A type of arthritis caused by psoriasis.

psychogenic: Caused by or related to psychological/emotional disorders.

psychological: Relating to behavior or the processes of the mind.

psychosis: A severe mental disorder in which there is a loss of reality and an inability to think clearly.

psychosomatic: Describes physical signs and symptoms that are influenced by psychological factors.

psychotherapy: Medical treatment of emotional disorders.

ptosis: Drooping of the upper eyelid.

pulmonary: Referring to or associated with the lungs.

pulp: A soft tissue mass such as the pads of the fingers; the soft tissue inside a tooth containing blood vessels and nerves.

pulsed current: Regular intervals of electrical currents that are packaged into groups of three or more pulses.

pulsed ultrasound: The use of ultrasound in which there are intermittent on and off cycles so as to reduce the thermal effects.

pupil: The portion of the iris that controls the amount of light that enters the eye by constricting or dilating.

purpura: Small hemorrhages causing purplish spots on the skin.

purulent: Pus-containing infection.

pus: A thick, yellowish fluid containing bacteria and necrotic white blood cells.

pustule: A small blister containing pus.

pyelolithotomy: Surgical removal of a kidney stone.

pyelonephritis: A bacterial infection causing inflammation of the kidney.

pyloric sphincter: The circular muscle between the stomach and small intestine that controls the passage of food.

Q

Q-angle: Quadriceps angle. The angle that is created at the knee by the intersection of a line along the patellar tendon (tibial tubercle to midpoint of the patella) and a line along the femur (from the ASIS to the midpoint of the patella). Normal Q-angle is 13° for males and 18° for females.

quadriplegia: Partial or complete loss of motor and sensory function of all four limbs.

qualitative research: An approach to measurement that is more subjective or judgmental.

quantitative research: An approach to measurement that is more objective.

quinapril (Accupril): An ACE inhibitor.

radial nerve: One of the terminal branches of the brachial plexus arising from the nerve roots C5-T1. It passes posteriorly and supplies sensation to the posterior upper arm and innervates the muscles of the posterior upper arm and radial side of the posterior arm.

radiating pain: Pain that emanates from a pathology and often follows the path of a nerve.

radiation: Energy traveling in the form of waves; a method of electromagnetic (including heat) transfer in which no medium is required.

radiation therapy: A radioactive treatment for diseases such as cancer that attacks the targeted tissue cells.

radical mastectomy: A treatment for breast cancer in which the entire breast, pectoral muscles, lymph nodes, and other tissues are removed.

radical surgery: Extreme or drastic measures, often a final resort; the surgical removal of tissue affected by disease.

radiculitis: *See* radiculopathy.

radiculopathy: Disorder of the spinal nerve root; radiating pain that follows a nerve distribution.

radiography (x-ray): A diagnostic procedure in which images of the inside of the body are formed using a form of radiation that is projected through the body and onto film.

radius: One of the long bones of the arm, it is the bone located on the thumb side. When the arm is in anatomical position, it sits lateral to the ulna.

ramipril (Altrace): An ACE inhibitor.

randomization: The selection of sample groups in which each member of the population has equal opportunity of being selected.

range of motion (ROM): The motion available at a joint in each plane, measured in degrees.

rapid eye movement (REM): The stage of deep sleep in which the eyes are moving.

rate of rise: Related to the shape of a waveform. It is a measure of how quickly the impulse rises from 0 to peak amplitude.

rating of perceived exertion (RPE): *See* Borg scale.

ratio scales: A measurement scale based on order in which there are equal units between measures and a base of zero. Examples include force, distance, number of repetitions, and time.

Raynaud's disease: A condition of unknown cause in which there is a vasospasm of the blood vessels supplying the fingers and toes, causing them to become pale, numb, and painful when exposed to cold.

reaction time: The time from stimulus to reaction.

rearfoot valgus: A structural malalignment of calcaneal eversion. May contribute to pes planus and excessive pronation.   Also called hindfoot valgus.

rearfoot varus: A structural malalignment of calcaneal inversion. May contribute to pes cavus and may contribute to excessive supination, leading to a multitude of overuse lower leg and foot injuries (eg, medial tibial stress syndrome; plantar fasciitis; and other knee, hip, and ankle injuries). Also called hindfoot varus.

receptive field: An area supplied by a given nerve.

receptor: A sensory nerve ending; nerve cell that responds to a stimulus; specialized sensory cells that detect chemical, mechanical, thermal, and other changes; *See also* mechanoreceptor, proprioceptor.

reciprocal inhibition: A reflex relaxation of the antagonist muscle group upon agonist contraction.

rectilinear: The path of movement along a straight line.

rectum: The distal end of the large intestine connecting the large intestine to the anus.

rectus femoris tightness test: *See* Kendall test.

recumbent: Lying down.

reduction of fracture: A procedure to realign the ends of a fracture; may be performed closed (no surgery) or open (surgical procedure).

referred pain: Pain in an area other than the site of injury or illness. Example: Kerr's sign is pain in the left shoulder caused by injury or illness to the spleen.

reflex: An involuntary activity involving simple circuitry from which a stimulus causes an automatic reaction such as the automatic withdrawal of the hand from a source of heat. *See also* deep tendon reflex.

reflex sympathetic dystrophy (RSD): Pain disproportionate or delayed recovery not consistent with the severity of injury. Signs and symptoms include hypersensitivity, decreased strength, spasm, edema, and dermatologic changes.

regeneration: The process of repair, regrowth, or restoration of a tissue following injury.

rehydration: A process of restoring the normal water, sodium, glucose, and electrolyte levels of the body.

Reiter's syndrome: A common reactive arthritic condition; an inflammation disorder affecting one or more joints, the urethra, and sometimes the conjunctiva.

relapse: The return of symptoms following a period of improvement.

relative refractory period: The period following depolarization when the membrane is "repolarizing," in which an action potential could occur if stimulus of sufficient strength (greater than that required to reach threshold when at rest) is applied.

reliability: A measure of the consistency of the data.

relocation test: A test for shoulder anterior apprehension in which the examiner applies a posterior force to the apprehensive patient during the anterior apprehension test. A reduction in apprehension is a positive sign.

REM: *See* rapid eye movement.

remission: The time in which there is a disappearance of a disease or its symptoms.

renal: Nephric; referring to the kidney.

renal cell carcinoma: A common type of kidney cancer.

renal colic: Severe pain in a kidney caused by a kidney stone.

repetitive strain injury: An injury that occurs when the same movement is repeated continuously. Common repetitive strain injuries include carpal tunnel syndrome and medial tibial stress syndrome.

residual: Something that lingers or remains; a permanent condition that results from an injury or illness.

residual volume: The air that remains in the lungs after a forcible exhalation (approximately 60 to 100 cubic inches).

resistance: A force applied against another force; the opposition to the flow of electrical current, measured in ohms; electrical impedance.

resistive force: A force that resists the motion caused by a motive force. When lifting a weight against gravity, the muscles provide the motive force while gravity provides a resistive force. When lowering a weight with gravity, gravity provides the motive force, while the muscles provide a resistive force.

respiratory arrest: The absence of breathing.

respiratory distress syndrome: A life-threatening condition in which an individual is unable to breath normally caused by injury or illness leading to a decrease in oxygen to the tissues.

respiratory failure: An increase in carbon dioxide and decrease in oxygen in the blood caused by the failure of the body to adequately exchange gases.

resting pulse: The normal pulse rate expected of an individual while at rest (80 bpm in adults).

retina: The light sensitive portion of the eye that contains the rods and cones.

retinaculum: A dense, fibrous retaining band that acts to hold tendons in place.

retinopathy: A disease of the retina most commonly a consequence of hypertension or diabetes mellitus.

retraction: Adduction of the scapula.

retro: Denoting backward or behind.

retrograde: Moving backward; retrograde amnesia is the inability to remember details prior to the onset of injury or illness.

retroversion: Of the hip, it refers to external rotation.

Reye's syndrome: A rare disorder mainly affecting children and teens, characterized by vomiting, disorientation, lethargy, and liver damage following a viral infection. May be linked to the use of aspirin in the treatment of viral infection.

rhabdomyolysis: A serious and sometimes fatal condition of renal failure due to the by-products of severe skeletal muscle trauma. Other causes include drugs, chemical reaction, septic shock. Traumatic rhabdomyolysis is also called crush syndrome.

rheo: Electrical current; blood flow.

rheobase: The minimum current required to reach tissue excitation when maximum phase duration is used.

rheumatoid arthritis: A chronic, systemic, inflammatory disease of the joints, particularly the fingers, wrists, feet, ankles, hips, knees, and shoulders; can also affect other joints such as costovertebral, sternoclavicular, etc. Diagnosed by the presence of rheumatoid factor in the blood.

rheumatoid factors: The presence of antibodies in individuals with rheumatoid arthritis (only 80% of individuals with rheumatoid arthritis test positive for rheumatoid factors).

rhinitis: Inflammation of the nasal passage causing congestion, sneezing, and runny nose, caused by the common cold or allergies (allergic rhinitis).

rhythmic stabilization: A type of proprioceptive neuromuscular facilitation technique that involves isometric cocontractions of opposing muscle groups. The patient contracts and "holds" against the practitioner's alternating force against the antagonist and then agonist muscle groups.

rickets: *See* osteomalacia.

right rotation: A rotation of the trunk or neck toward the right.

rigidity: In a muscle, resistance to movement throughout the range of motion; abdominal rigidity caused by muscle guarding is often a sign of internal bleeding and injury to an organ. *Decerebrate*—indicating brainstem injury; extension and adduction of the upper extremity joints; and extension, internal rotation, and plantar flexion in the lower extremity. *Decorticate*—Indicating injury above the brainstem, flexion and adduction of the upper extremity joints, extension, internal rotation, and plantar flexion in the lower extremity.

ringworm: Tinea; a highly contagious fungal infection of the skin that can be spread by direct contact; appears as a red scaly circle; common in wrestling.

Rinne's test: A test that utilizes a tuning fork to determine if hearing loss is due to perception or conduction. The tuning fork is held in the air near the ear and then placed on the mastoid bone. If the sound is heard longer when the tuning fork is held in the air, the test is positive for perception loss. If the sound is heard longer when the tuning fork is in contact with the mastoid, the test is negative and indicates conduction loss.

RNA (ribonucleic acid): Found in all cells; concerned with protein synthesis.

Rocky mountain spotted fever: A rare disease transmitted to humans by ticks; signs and symptoms include fever, muscle pain, and a spreading red rash. Treated with antibiotics. Untreated, the disease may be fatal.

roentenogram: X-ray.

Rolfing: A type of therapeutic massage involving soft tissue manipulation with the intent of balancing the body within a gravitational field.

Romberg's sign: A test for neurological dysfunction in which the patient stands with eyes open and arms to the side. The patient then closes his or her eyes and the examiner notes disturbances in balance. Modified Romberg's sign is performed on a single limb to assess neuromuscular control and somatosensory input from the lower extremity (especially the foot).

Roo's test: A special test of the shoulder specifically for thoracic outlet syndrome. *See* Special Tests—Shoulder (Appendix 17).

rosacea: A skin disease affecting adults (usually 30 to 50 years old) characterized by chronic redness on the forehead, cheeks, chin, and nose caused by dilated blood vessels.

rotation: Motion that follows a circular path and takes place about an axis.

rotator cuff: A structure made up of the SITS (supraspinatus, infraspinatus, teres minor, subscapularis) muscles that in addition to rotation of the shoulder play an important role in the stability of the shoulder joint.

rubella: German measles; an acute, mild infection caused by the rubella virus. Signs and symptoms include rash and fever. Can cause birth defects when a woman is infected during the early stages of pregnancy.

runner's knee: *See* iliotibial band (ITB) friction syndrome.

rupture: A break or tear in a tissue.

sacral apex: A special test of the sacroiliac joint. *See* Special Tests—Hip (Appendix 17).

sacral plexus: A network of nerves made up of nerve roots S1-4 that blend and divide to form a network.

sacroiliac: The joint between the ilium of the pelvis and the sacrum.

sacroiliitis: Inflammation of the sacroiliac joints.

sacrum: The broad, spade-shaped bone located at the bottom of the spine forming the posterior wall of the pelvis. The sacrum is formed by the fusion of five sacral vertebrae.

SAD: *See* seasonal affective disorder.

sagittal: A vertical plane passing through the body from front to back. The midsagittal plane divides the body into left and right halves.

sagittal plane: Midsaggital; divides the body into left and right parts. Motions that take place in this plane include flexion/extension.

sag test: *See* profile test.

SAID principle: Abbreviation for "specific adaptation to imposed demands;" the body will adapt to whatever increased demands are placed on it; related to the overload principle.

saline: A solution that contains 0.9% sodium chloride.

sarcoidosis: Besnier-Boeck-Schaumann disease; a rare systemic disease of unknown cause consisting of inflammation and fibrosis especially of the lungs, but also in the lymph nodes, liver, skin, glands, and eyes.

sarcoma: A type of connective tissue cancer, usually highly malignant.

Saturday night palsy: Temporary paralysis of the arm after extended pressure on the nerves in the axilla. The name is derived from the situation when one "passes out" in a position where there will be pressure on the axilla (and the nerves in the brachial plexus) for an extended period. The axillary nerve or radial nerve is commonly affected, leading to the temporary inability to abduct the shoulder or extend the elbow.

scabies: A highly contagious skin disorder caused by mites. The female mite burrows into the skin producing an intensely itchy vesicular eruption.

scalenectomy: The surgical removal of one or more of the scalene muscles.

scaphoid: Navicular of the hand; the most lateral bone in the first (proximal) layer of carpals. A common site of nonunion in fractures due to poor blood supply.

scapula: The large, flat, triangular bone of the shoulder girdle that sits posterior and lateral over the ribs. The lateral angle of the scapula forms the glenoid fossa that articulates with the humerus and lies just superior to the acromion process that articulates with the clavicle.

scapulohumeral: Relating to the scapula and humerus.

scapulohumeral rhythm: The relationship between glenohumeral motion and scapular motion during shoulder abduction, commonly reported as a 2:1 ratio. The ratio is actually much more complex than this. In the first 30 degrees of motion, there is little scapular motion. McQuade & Smidt (1998) reported approximately 8:1 ratio at the beginning of motion reducing to a 2:1 ratio near the end of ROM during passive movement. AROM with a heavy load changed the ratio significantly. With a heavy load, at the beginning of ROM, the ratio was approximately 2:1, but near the end the ratio increased to 4.5:1.

Scheuermann's disease (juvenile kyphosis): An adolescent skeletal disease that results in a hunched back.

schizophrenia: A type of psychosis characterized by distorted perception, abnormal thought processes, and personality disorders, including split or multiple personalities.

sciatica: Pain along the sciatic nerve most commonly caused by nerve root compression or piriformis syndrome.

sclera: The tough, white portion of the eye.

scleroderma: A painful hardening and contraction of the connective tissues; can remain localized or may spread to other tissues; can result in death.

scoliosis: A congenital or acquired abnormal lateral deviation of the vertebral column, commonly "S" or "C" shaped.

screening: A process of evaluating an otherwise healthy person in order to detect potential abnormalities. Preseason or preparticipation screening is common prior to the start of an athletic season.

seasonal affective disorder (SAD): A psychological, emotional disorder characterized by depression brought on by the change of season (particularly fall and winter) and shorter days.

sebaceous cyst: A cyst (closed sac or pouch) of an oil secreting gland (including hair follicles) of the skin. Also called epidermoid cysts.

seborrhea: Excessive secretion of sebum (oil) on the face and scalp.

sebum: An oily secretion from the sebaceous glands.

secondary: Not primary; describes a disease or injury caused by another one (primary).

secondary cell death: Death of the cells due to lack of oxygen secondary to edema.

secondary motion: Also called accessory motion. The small motions of sliding, spinning, and rolling that are necessary in order to have physiological (primary) motion.

secondary oocyte: The larger of two ovums following the first division of meiosis.

secondary survey: Patient assessment that occurs following a primary survey when there are no immediate life-threatening conditions. Secondary survey includes respiratory rate, heart rate, observation of skin color and temperature, observation for bleeding, discoloration, fractures, etc.

second-class lever: Is a type of machine in which the resistive force is between the axis and motive forces. Examples include a wheel barrow and a nut cracker. Most eccentric actions in the body are performed by second-class levers due to the force of gravity acting as the motive force during an eccentric contraction. The advantage of this type of lever arrangement is that the motive force always has a longer level arm and thus, a greater force advantage in producing an equal torque.

second impact syndrome: A head injury, sometimes apparently very mild, that occurs before the symptoms of a previous head injury have resolved. This is a very serious injury with a mortality rate of 50%.

second order neuron: Afferent neurons in the spinal cord or brain.

sedative: A pharmacologic agent that has a calming effect used to relieve anxiety, tension, and insomnia.

seizure: Sudden electrical hyperactivity in the brain, causing loss of consciousness or convulsions.

sepsis: Destruction of tissue by bacteria; can result in an infection in which bacteria is dangerously spread into the bloodstream.

septic arthritis: Inflammatory joint disease caused by a bacterial infection.

septicemia: Also known as blood poisoning; an invasion of microorganisms into the blood stream caused by infection often accompanied by abscess and toxemic symptoms.

septic shock: A severe and life threatening consequence of sepsis in which blood pressure drops due to blood poisoning.

sequela: The result or consequence of a previous injury or disorder.

sequestration: A severe type of disk herniation in which the disk fragments into small pieces.

serotonin: A neurotransmitter important to sleep and a chemical mediator thought to play a role in the inflammatory process.

sesamoid: Small round bone or cartilage in a tendon that acts to increase leverage by increasing the angle of pull of the tendon (eg, patella).

Sever's disease: Calcaneal apophysitis.

sharpened Romberg: A variation of Romberg's sign in which the patient stands with one foot directly in front of the other (heel to toe).

shear: The movement of one surface over another within the same plane of motion.

shingles: *See* herpes zoster.

shin splints: A generic term for "shin pain" or medial tibial stress syndrome.

shock: A result of circulatory collapse caused by severe bleeding, cardiac or respiratory distress, allergic reaction, pain, or emotional distress. Can become life-threatening without treatment.

shortwave diathermy: A deep heating modality from the electromagnetic spectrum that uses high frequency electromagnetic energy. Shortwave diathermy has wavelengths ranging from 11 to 22 m and operates at a frequency of approximately 13 to 27 MHz.

shunt: A passageway (congenital or artificial) that channels or diverts blood from one area to another.

sickle cell anemia: A hereditary disease affecting African Americans in which red blood cells have a characteristic "sickling" (oblong shape). These cells cease to be circulated, causing anemia.

side effect: An unwanted consequence of a treatment.

sigmoidoscopy: The use of a scope to examine the rectum and the large intestine.

sign: A characteristic of a disease or injury that is observed by the examiner and may or may not have been noticed by the patient (compare to symptom).

significance: A statistical term that is used to describe a difference in mean scores or a relationship that is not due simply to chance.

sign of buttock: A special test for tumor or trochanteric bursitis. *See* Special Tests—Hip (Appendix 17).

silver fork fracture: A Colles' fracture in which the profile appears to take on the shape of a fork.

sinusitis: Inflammation of the sinuses, usually as a result of a bacterial infection.

sinus rhythm: Normal heart rhythm.

SLAP lesion: Injury to the Superior Labrum with Anterior Posterior instability. O'Brien's is a test for SLAP lesion.

sleep apnea: A condition in which there is a temporary cessation of breathing during sleep.

sling psychrometer: A measurement device to determine relative humidity by reading a "wet" bulb and "dry" bulb.

slipped capital femoral epiphysis: A posterior or inferior slippage of the femoral head seen most commonly in boys age 10 to 17.

slipped disk: *See* disk injury or prolapse.

slow twitch fiber: *See* type I fiber.

slump test: Special test for the presence of spinal cord, dura, or nerve root injury in which the patient is seated with one knee extended and the trunk flexed while the examiner passively flexes the neck.

Smith's fracture: A reverse Colles' fracture in which the displacement is toward the palmar side.

Snellen's chart: A chart used to assess visual acuity that has printed letters that decrease in size on each subsequent line.

soft tissue mobilization: *See* myofascial release.

solar plexus: The largest plexus in the body, located behind the stomach.

soma: Cell body.

somatic: Pertaining to the body.

spasm: An involuntary abnormal muscular contraction.

spasticity: Muscle stiffness and resistance that gives way to increased passive movement. *See also* spastic paralysis.

spastic paralysis: Spasticity or increased reflex activity with concomitant weakness of the limbs caused by disease of the corticospinal tract. *See also* spasticity.

Speeds test: A special test of the shoulder to determine the presence of biceps tendonitis or biceps tendon subluxation. *See* Special Tests—Shoulder (Appendix 17).

spermatic cord torsion: An injury to the testicle, usually a direct blow, causing the testicles to revolve in the scrotum producing pain, nausea, vomiting, and inflammation; can lead to atrophy. Physician referral is recommended.

sphygmomanometer: The measurement instrument used to assess blood pressure.

spica: A figure-8 type wrapping procedure around a joint.

spina bifida: A birth defect in which there is a failure of the spine to fuse, leaving the spine underdeveloped and exposed. There are various degrees of this deformity.

spina bifida occulta: The least severe form of spina bifida, in which there is no protrusion of the spinal cord or its membrane.

spinal fusion: A surgical procedure in which two or more adjacent vertebrae are joined using bone fragments or surgical hardware to treat spinal instability.

spine of the scapula: The nearly horizontal bone across the dorsum of the scapula above which sits the supraspinatus muscle and below which sits the infraspinatus muscle. The lateral end of the spine of the scapula forms the acromion process (point of the shoulder).

spirometer: A gasometer that measures respiratory gases; device to measure lung capacity by measuring the volume of air exhaled.

spleen: An organ located in the upper left quadrant of the abdomen whose function is to produce lymphocytes and store red blood cells.

splenectomy: Surgical removal of the spleen.

splint: A device that is used to immobilize a body part.

spondylitis: Inflammation of the synovial joints of the vertebrae.

spondylolisis: A defect in the pars interarticularis of the vertebra known as a "collared Scottie dog."

spondylolisthesis: A defect in the pars interarticularis of the vertebra with a forward slippage of the vertebral body known as a "decapitated Scottie dog."

spoon-shaped nails: A condition that causes the nails to curl up forming a "spoon-shape." A symptom of anemia, iron deficiency, diabetes, psoriasis, or congenital abnormality.

SPORTDiscuss: A bibliographic database, international in scope, covering all aspects of sport, fitness, recreation, and related fields. Articles from more than 2000 sport-related journals, monographs, articles, books, theses, and CD-ROMs in English, French, and other languages are indexed for inclusion. The Sport Information Resource Center (SIRC), the database provider, is the largest resource center in the world collecting and disseminating information in the area of sport, physical education, physical fitness, and sports medicine.

sprain: To stretch or tear a ligament, the fibrous connective tissue that attaches bone to bone.

Sprengel's deformity: Congenital elevation of the scapula.

Spurling's test: Special test of the cervical spine for nerve root compression. *See* Special Tests—Spine (Appendix 17).

sputum: Saliva and mucus that is coughed up from the lungs and airway.

squinting patella: Medially facing, rotated patella caused by femoral medial torsion (anteversion) or tibial lateral torsion.

squish test: Special test of the sacroiliac joint. *See* Special Tests—Hip (Appendix 17).

standard deviation: A measure of how spread out the observed scores are from their mean.

standard error of the mean: The amount of error in the prediction of the true (population) mean.

standardized test: A test that has been developed and tested, has established procedures and norms, and demonstrated reliability and validity.

staphylococci: A gram-positive bacteria that causes skin infections and other purulent infections.

stasis: A slowing or blockage of the normal flow of fluid.

stenosis: Abnormal narrowing of a passage.

step deformity: A deformity caused by acromioclavicular separation.

sternum: The long, flat bone central to the thorax articulating with the clavicle and the cartilage of the ribs, made up of the manubrium, body, and xiphoid process.

steroids: Fat soluble organic compounds naturally occurring or synthetic. The naturally occurring steroids include androgen, estrogen, progesterone, bile salts, and sterols. Synthetic steroids include corticosteroids and anabolic steroids. Corticosteroids include cortisone, hydrocortisone, and corticosterone, which have powerful anti-inflammatory effects, while aldosterone is used primarily for the regulation of sodium and water. Anabolic steroids include ethylestranol, methandienone, nandrolone, norethandrolone, oxymesterone, and stanalone. They have been linked to serious side effects including depression, hostility, suicide, liver damage, other severe health disorders, and death.

stinger: *See* neurapraxia.

stoma: Mouth; an artificial opening created surgically.

strabismus: Abnormal alignment of the eyes, such as heterotropia when one eye looks upward and one downward, or crossed eyes.

strain: A stretch or tear in a muscle or tendon; the deformation of an object; *See also* stress-strain curve (expressed as units of force x length or joules).

strength: A measure of a muscle's ability to exert a maximal force against a resistance.

strength-duration curve: A graphical illustration of the relationship between the duration of an electrical current and the strength (intensity) of the current needed to reach an action potential. As the duration is increased, less intensity is required to achieve the same result.

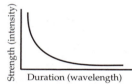

strep throat: Streptococcus bacteria causing sore throat, fever, and swollen lymph nodes.

streptococci: Gram-positive bacteria that cause a variety of diseases, including scarlet fever, pneumonia, and strep throat.

stress: An internal force divided by the area over which it is applied. Expressed in Newtons/m^2 or pascals.

stress fracture: Also called fatigue fracture; a fracture caused by repetitive motions such as running, marching, etc.

stress-strain curve: A plot of the relationship of stress to strain (the elastic modulus) of a material.

stretch-shortening exercise: *See* plyometric.

stroke: Apoplexy; a sudden interruption of blood flow to the brain causing loss of consciousness, sensation, and movement. Damage to the brain due to lack of blood supply (from blockage in an artery) or rupture of a blood vessel leads to complete or partial loss of function in the area of the body that is controlled by that portion of the brain. Severity varies greatly.

stye: Bacterial infection causing inflammation in the follicle of an eyelash.

subacute: Condition that appears just beyond and is less severe than the acute stage.

subcutaneous: Below the cutaneous layer (skin).

subdural hematoma: Bleeding in the brain below the dura matter, usually venous bleeding with slower onset of symptoms (could be as long as 24 hours to 1 month). Compare to epidural hematoma.

subjective measure: A measure based on judgment of an individual (contrast to objective).

subluxation: A partial or incomplete dislocation, or a dislocation followed by an immediate and spontaneous relocation.

substance P: A neurotransmitter thought to play an important role in initiation of transmission of an impulse along a first order neuron and at the synapse between first order and second order neurons.

substantia gelatinosa: An area in the dorsal horn of the spinal cord thought to play an important role in the control of pain. *See also* gate control theory.

substitution: The improper use of other muscles to perform an activity. The use of substitute motions can promote incorrect motor programming and dysfunction.

subtalar: Below the talus; the articulation between the talus and calcaneus.

sudden death syndrome: A general term used to describe unexpected sudden cardiac death in young individuals.

sudden infant death syndrome (SIDS): The unexpected death of an otherwise healthy baby; the cause is unknown.

sulcus sign: A special test of the shoulder to assess glenohumeral instability. *See* Special Tests—Shoulder (Appendix 17).

superficial: On top, near the surface, shallow.

superior: Above.

supination (of the arm): External rotation of the forearm so as to place the palm up.

supination (of the foot): The act of turning upward; in the foot, supination is dependent upon whether the motion is performed open or closed chain. During closed chain movement, supination involves dorsiflexion, inversion, and abduction. During open chain movement, supination involves plantar flexion, inversion, and adduction.

supine: With the back or dorsal surface downward; lying face up.

suprascapular nerve: The nerve supplying the supraspinatus and infraspinatus.

sural: Relating to the leg (lower leg).

suture: Surgical closure of a wound; an immovable joint such as the sutures of the skull.

swan neck deformity: A deformity of the finger(s) in which the metacarpophalangeal joint and distal interphalangeal joints are flexed while the proximal interphalangeal joint is hyperextended.

sway index: An indirect measure of balance or postural sway, it is the standard deviation of time and distance the individual spent away from his or her center of balance. The Chattecx Dynamic Balance System (Chattanooga Group Inc) uses the sway index.

swimmer's ear: *See* otitis externa.

swing phase: The phase during a walking cycle between toe off and heel strike.

symmetrical: The same; similar bilaterally.

symptom (Sx): A characteristic of a disease or injury that is experienced and described by the patient (compare to sign).

synapse: The act of an electrical nerve impulse crossing from one neuron to the next; the gap between two neurons (synaptic cleft).

syncope: Fainting, loss of consciousness due to insufficient blood flow to the brain.

syndrome: A group of signs and symptoms that when found together are characteristics of a particular disorder.

synergist: A muscle that "assists" an agonist; a drug interaction that together produces a desired effect that each drug would not produce if given alone.

synovectomy: Surgical removal of a synovial membrane.

synovial fluid: A viscous fluid secreted by the synovial membrane found in synovial joints, tendon sheaths, and bursa.

synovial membrane: The thin mesothelium and connective tissue membrane that encloses a moveable joint and secretes synovial fluid.

synovitis: Inflammation of the synovial membrane. Signs and symptoms include redness, swelling, joint stiffness, and pain. Common causes are rheumatoid arthritis or infection.

synthesis: The union of chemical elements so as to form a whole.

syphilis: Sexually transmitted disease with symptoms that appear within 10 days to 2 months after contact. Papulae on the genitals develop into ulcers (chancre) that are highly contagious. Fever, headache, and body rash can occur in later stages. Antibiotic treatment is necessary to prevent serious effects on organs of the body.

systemic: Affecting the whole body.

systemic lupus erythematosus: An autoimmune inflammatory connective tissue disease of unknown cause in which fever, rash, arthritis, anemia, and hemorrhages in the skin and mucous membranes occur. In more serious cases, inflammation of the pericardium and damage to the kidneys and central nervous system can occur.

systolic pressure: Blood pressure measured while the heart is contracting; the normal systolic pressure in an adult is 120 mmHg, normal diastolic pressure is 80 mmHg, recorded as 120/80 mmHg.

T

tachycardia: A fast heart rate, usually over 100 beats per minute in adults.

talar tilt: A special test of the ankle to assess the medial and lateral ligaments. *See* Special Tests—Foot/Ankle (Appendix 17).

talipes equinovarus: Clubfoot; weight-bearing occurs on the ball of the foot and lateral aspect of the foot.

tapotement: A massage technique involving percussion of "cupped" hands.

tarsal tunnel syndrome: Tibial nerve compression as it crosses the ankle medially deep to the flexor retinaculum and tibiocalcaneal ligament through the tarsal tunnel.

T cell: *See* T-lymphocyte.

temporomandibular joint syndrome (TMJ): A disorder of the temporomandibular joint causing headache and tenderness of the jaw and teeth.

tendinitis: Inflammation of a tendon.

tendon: A strong, fibrous connective tissue that connects muscle to bone.

tendon transfer: The repositioning of a tendon for the purpose of redefining the role of the muscle and/or tendon.

tennis elbow: *See* lateral epicondylitis.

tenosynovitis: Inflammation of the synovial sheath of a tendon.

tensile: Referring to tension.

tensiometer: A device designed to measure the amount of tension or force applied.

testicular torsion: Severe pain and swelling of a testicle due to twisting of the spermatic cord.

testosterone: A male sex hormone produced in the testes in males and in the adrenal cortex in males and females; responsible for the development of male secondary sex characteristics.

tetanus: A sometimes fatal disease characterized by painful tonic muscular contractions caused by bacteria present in soil and manure. The DTaP vaccine is given at 2, 4, 6, 15 months, and 4 to 6 years. Persons receiving all five doses may not require booster until age 50. Most adults have not, and thus should receive a booster every 10 years.

tetracycline: One of the antibiotic drugs used to treat a variety of infections.

thenar: The thumb side of the "heel of the hand."

therapeutic range: The range of dosage of a treatment modality or drug that will produce the desired effects without the unwanted side effects.

thermotherapy: A therapeutic modality involving the use of heat.

third-class lever: A type of machine in which the motive force is between the axis and resistive forces. Examples include a snow shovel, an oar, and a baseball bat. In the body, most joint movements are performed by third-class levers. The advantages of a third-class lever are speed of movement and range of motion. A distinct disadvantage is that the motive force will always have a shorter lever arm, thus requiring a greater amount of force to produce the same amount of torque.

third-order neuron: Afferent neurons in the brain.

Thomas test: A special test of the hip to assess hip flexion contracture. *See* Special Tests—Hip (Appendix 17).

Thompson's test: A special test of the Achille's tendon to assess for rupture. *See* Special Tests—Foot/Ankle (Appendix 17).

thoracic outlet syndrome (TOS): A condition in which the brachial plexus and/or subclavian artery become stretched or more likely, impinged, causing radiating pain, numbness (neurogenic symptoms), and reduced circulation (vascular symptoms). Common causes are scalene muscles, cervical rib anomaly, depressed shoulder, and poor posture. In over 90% of cases, there are no vascular symptoms.

thoracodorsal nerve: The nerve supplying the latissimus dorsi, it arises from C6-8 and the posterior trunk of the brachial plexus.

thorax: The chest.

threshold: The point above which a reaction will take place and below which no reaction will occur. Threshold must be met in order to reach an action potential. Once threshold is met, there is complete depolarization (all or none response).

thrombectomy: Removal of a blood clot.

thrombocytopenic purpura: An abnormally small number of platelets in the blood, causing abnormal bruising due to bleeding.

thromboembolism: An obstruction caused by a thrombus (clot) that has dislodged and traveled from another area.

thrombophlebitis: Inflammation of a vein with concomitant clot formation in the affected area.

thrombosis: The formation of a blood clot within a vessel.

thrombus: A blood clot.

thyroid gland: A gland located posterior and lateral to the larynx responsible for the secretion of thyroid hormone and calcitonin.

thyroiditis: Inflammation of the thyroid gland.

tibia: The large weightbearing bone of the lower leg.

tibial nerve: One of the branches of the sciatic nerve that extends posterior along the back of the leg below the knee and supplies the muscles of the posterior leg.

tibial stress: *See* medial tibial stress syndrome.

tibial torsion: Excessive rotation of the tibia.

Tietze's syndrome: A painful condition in which there is inflammation of the costocartilage.

tinea: A skin fungus, typically ringworm.

tinea capitis: A fungus of the scalp.

tinea corporis: An infection on the body area caused by a fungus.

tinea cruris: Also known as jock itch; an infection in the groin area caused by a fungus.

tinea pedis: Also known as athlete's foot; an infection of the foot caused by a fungus.

tinea versicolor: A skin fungus exhibiting yellow or light brown patches.

Tinel's sign: A special test for the presence of nerve injury or dysfunction in which the examiner "taps" over a superficial nerve such as the ulnar nerve in the ulnar groove, the median nerve in the carpal tunnel, the common peroneal as it wraps around the head of the fibula, or the tibial nerve as it crosses posterior to the medial malleolus. A normal "twinge" or brief tingling sensation is a negative test.

tinnitus: Ringing in the ears.

tissue hypoxia: Lack of oxygen to the tissues.

T-lymphocyte: A class of lymphocytes (white blood cells that fight infection) that originate from lymphoid stem cells and migrate from the bone marrow to the thymus. T-lymphocytes help facilitate antibody production and assist in recognizing and rejecting foreign tissues. Uncontrolled proliferation can cause T-cell leukemia/lymphoma.

toe-off: The point following midstance when the weight is transferred to the toes and just before the foot leaves the ground.

tone: The normal tension of a relaxed muscle.

tonic (clonic): An unremitting muscular contraction.

tonsillectomy: The surgical removal of the tonsils.

tonsillitis: Inflammation of the tonsils.

tonsils: Any group of lymphoid tissue. Commonly we refer to the tonsils as the lymphoid tissue located bilaterally in the back of the throat.

torque: The product of force times distance. All rotary motions produce torque. In joint motions, torque is the product of muscular force times the perpendicular distance from the line of the force's action to the axis of rotation.

torque arm: *See* force arm.

torsion: Twisting action; tibial torsion is a rotation of the tibia about the longitudinal axis relative to the position of the femur; femoral torsion is a rotation of the femur about the longitudinal axis relative to the position of the tibia.

torticollis: A cervical muscle spasm causing pain, stiffness, and a characteristic lateral flexion of the neck.

tourniquet: A device that encircles a limb that is used to temporarily stop the flow of blood or control bleeding to a distal body segment.

toxemia: The presence of toxic levels of bacteria in the blood.

toxic shock syndrome: An acute and sudden staphylococcus disease associated with the use of tampons, characterized by nausea, vomiting, erythema, and shock; sometimes fatal.

trachea: The hollow organ that connects the larynx to the two bronchi of the lungs.

tracheitis: Inflammation of the trachea.

tracheotomy: An opening created directly into the trachea in which a tube is inserted to facilitate respiration.

traction: The use of longitudinal tension to realign body segments.

transcutaneous: Through the skin.

transcutaneous electrical nerve stimulator (TENS): The use of electrical current to cause excitation of the nerves for the purposes of pain control. *See* gate control theory.

transducer: A device that transforms one type of energy into another, such as an ultrasound device that transforms electrical energy into a mechanical sound wave.

transferrin: An iron-transporting protein.

transient ischemic attack (TIA): A mini stroke, often a precursor to cerebrovascular accident. It is a temporary loss of blood supply to the brain causing temporary facial paralysis, numbness, slurred speech, and vision impairment.

transitory paralysis: Temporary paralysis.

transmissible: Referring to disease that can be passed from one person to another.

transplant: A surgical procedure in which an injured or ill organ is replaced with a healthy one.

transverse: A horizontal plane (parallel to the ground) passing through the body.

transverse arch: The arch formed perpendicular to the length of the foot, created by the cuneiforms, the cuboid, and the five metatarsals. The arch is strengthened by the interosseous, plantar, and dorsal ligaments as well as the adductor hallicus, the peroneus longus, and other interosseous muscles of the first and fifth toes.

transverse plane: Divides the body into upper and lower parts. Motions that take place in this plane include internal/external rotation, horizontal abduction/adduction, and trunk and neck rotation.

traumatic shock: Shock brought about by injury or surgery.

Trendelenburg's test: Special test of the hip for gluteus medius weakness. *See* Special Tests—Hip (Appendix 17).

triage: A process of classifying ill or injured individuals according to the severity of their conditions and the likelihood of survival.

triceps surae: The two heads of the gastrocnemius and the soleus.

tricuspid: The valve between the left atrium and ventricle.

trigeminal nerve: Cranial nerve V responsible for motor function involved in chewing and facial sensation. *See* Appendix 8.

trigeminal neuralgia: A condition affecting the fifth cranial nerve in which pain is present in the face and jaw.

trigger finger: In impairment, usually affecting the flexor tendon of the third or fourth finger. There is a thickening or a narrowing of the tendon sheath, causing the finger to "stick" in a flexed position when unclenching the fist, until suddenly it gives way as if someone released a trigger.

trigger point: A deep, tender, palpable area of tissue that when pressure is applied to it, causes the pattern of pain (sometimes radiating) to be reproduced.

triglyceride: A type of fat found in the blood related to increased incidence of heart disease, high blood pressure, and diabetes.

trochlear nerve: Cranial nerve IV responsible for eye movement along with the abducens and oculomotor nerves. *See* Appendix 8.

true leg length: Real leg length; a measurement from the medial malleolus to the ASIS.

t-test: A statistical test used to compare two sets of parametric data.

tuberculosis: An infectious bacterial disease of the lungs that is transmitted through the air.

tumor: An abnormal malignant or benign mass.

tunnel vision: A disease that causes loss of peripheral vision, commonly caused by glaucoma.

turf toe: A sprain of the first metatarsophalangeal joint.

two-point discrimination: The ability to discriminate fine cutaneous sensations. The examiner uses a two-point discriminator to determine the distance at which the patient can discriminate one point from two.

tympanic membrane: Eardrum.

type I diabetes: Also known as insulin-dependent diabetes mellitus or juvenile-onset diabetes; this is the more severe form, developing in childhood or adolescence and characterized by an inability to properly secrete insulin, causing hyperglycemia and potentially ketoacidosis.

type I error: The rejection of the null hypothesis when, in fact, the null is true.

type I fiber: Slow twitch fiber; slow oxidative fiber; takes twice as long as the fast twitch fibers to reach maximum tension but is more resistant to fatigue.

type II diabetes: Also called adult-onset noninsulin-dependent diabetes mellitus; this is the most common form of diabetes, characterized by hyperglycemia as a result of inadequate production and utilization of insulin.

type II error: Acceptance of the null hypothesis when, in fact, the null is false.

type II fiber: Fast twitch fiber; fast oxidative fiber; twice as fast as the type I at reaching maximum tension; capable of very quick, forceful contractions but fatigues quicker than type I.

U

ulcer: An open sore of the skin or mucous membrane, often referring to the lining of the stomach.

ulcerative colitis: Ulcers of the colon and rectum.

ulnar nerve: One of the terminal branches of the brachial plexus arising from the medial cord of the brachial plexus. The ulnar nerve crosses the elbow posteromedially through the ulnar groove and courses anteromedially along the ulnar side of the anterior forearm and supplies the medial palmar.

ultrasound: A therapeutic modality that uses sound waves.

ultrasound scanning: Sonography; the use of sound waves as a diagnostic process to view the internal organs.

ultraviolet (UV): An electromagnetic radiation that is beyond the visible light with a wavelength in the range of 180 to 390 nanometers. UV is used therapeutically to treat skin conditions.

umbilical hernia: A weak area in the abdominal wall, present at birth, in which the baby's intestines protrude through the wall near the umbilicus.

unilateral: Relating to only one side of the body.

universal precautions: A procedure for handling bodily fluids recommended by the Centers for Disease Control and Prevention in 1985 and updated in 1996. Refer to http://www.cdc.gov/niosh/topics/bbp/ or http://www.cdc. gov/for up-to-date information.

unsaturated fat: A type of fat or oil found mainly in vegetables.

upper-body ergometer (UBE): A device that measures the amount of work done by the upper extremities. Also called upper-body cycle.

upper motor neuron lesion (UMNL): Injury or illness in the corticospinal or pyramidal tract of the brain or spinal cord resulting in hemi-, para-, or quadriplegia. Symptoms include spasticity, paralysis, positive Babinski, and other pathological reflexes.

upper quarter screen: A quick check of the upper extremities to assist in localizing injury and to rule out gross neurological deficits. Includes cervical motions, shoulder girdle and shoulder joint motions, elbow, wrist, and hand motions, sensory and reflex assessment.

urea: Protein waste product that is created in the liver and released by the kidneys.

uremia: An abnormally high level of urea in the blood.

ureters: Bilateral tubes from the kidneys to the bladder.

urethra: The passageway from the bladder in which urine is released.

urethritis: Inflammation of the urethra.

urethrocele: A condition in which the urethra bulges into the vagina.

urethrocystitis: Inflammation of the urethra and the bladder.

urinalysis: Chemical assessment of the urine.

urinary incontinence: The inability to control the release of urine.

urinary tract: Includes the kidneys, ureters, bladder, and urethra.

uterus: The area in which the fetus develops following the fertilization of the egg.

uvea: The middle layer of the eye consisting of colored area just below the sclera.

uveitis: Inflammation of the uvea.

vaccination: A form of immunization in which antibodies to a particular disease are developed in the body in response to the introduction of a weakened form of a microorganism. The development of the antibodies will protect the body in the event that there is an exposure to the microorganisms.

vaginitis: Inflammation of the vagina characterized by itching and burning sensations.

vagus nerve: Cranial nerve X responsible for breathing; swallowing; and sensation of the larynx, pharynx, and bronchii. *See* Appendix 8.

valgus: A deformity in which the distal end of a bone deviates laterally, such as "knock knees;" also known as genu (knee) valgum.

valgus stress: The application of ligamentous stress applied to the lateral aspect of the limb forcing the limb into a valgus position.

validity: The soundness of a measurement technique to measure what it was intended to measure.

Valsalva's maneuver: A special test for nerve involvement. *See* Special Tests—Spine (Appendix 17).

variance: The average of the squared deviations from the mean.

varicella: Chickenpox.

varicocele: Varicose veins on the testicles.

varicose veins: Enlarged or inflamed veins near the surface of the skin, often causing discomfort or pain.

variola: Smallpox.

varus: A deformity in which the distal end of a bone deviates medially, such as "bowlegged;" also known as genu (knee) varum.

varus stress: The application of ligamentous stress applied to the medial aspect of the limb forcing the limb into a varus position.

vas deferens: A small passageway that stores and transports sperm.

vascular: Relating to blood vessels.

vasculitis: Inflammation of the blood vessels.

vasectomy: A surgical procedure in which the vas deferens are cut and tied off so that sperm will no longer be present in the semen; sterilization.

vasoconstriction: A process in which there is a narrowing of blood vessels.

vasodilation: A process in which there is an opening or widening of blood vessels.

vasospasm: A constriction of a blood vessel, reducing blood flow.

vasovagal attack: A sudden loss of consciousness due to a decrease in heart rate.

vein: A blood vessel responsible for carrying the blood back to the heart.

venereal disease (VD): Any sexually transmitted disease.

ventilator: An apparatus that provides breathing for a person who cannot breathe on his or her own.

ventral: Front, anterior.

ventricle: A chamber responsible for the circulation of fluid; the heart contains a left and right ventricle responsible for pumping blood through the body; the brain contains four chambers (ventricles) that contatin cerebrospinal fluid.

ventricular fibrillation: Irregular contractions of the heart in which the heart is "out of sync" and not effective in circulating blood.

verruca: Common wart; a rough benign growth of the skin caused by a virus. May disappear spontaneously.

verruca plantaris: Commonly called plantar warts; found on the soles of the feet. Due to the constant pressure of weight-bearing, plantar warts tend to grow in rather than protruding up as is the case with most warts. Eventually this causes a painful condition during weight-bearing and the wart must be removed.

verruca vulgaris: A wart that may occur anywhere but commonly found on dorsal aspect of hands and fingers.

vertebra: A small, irregular-shaped bone of the spine; there are 33 bones that make up the spine: 7 cervical, 12 thoracic, 5 lumbar, 5 sacral, and 4 coccygeal.

vertical: Upright; perpendicular to horizontal.

vertigo: Dizziness.

very low-density lipoprotein (VLDL): A blood protein that is associated with heart disease.

vesicle: A small, fluid-filled sac.

vestibulocochlear nerve: Cranial nerve VIII responsible for hearing and balance. *See* Appendix 8.

viral: Pertaining to a virus.

virus: A disease-causing microorganism that reproduces itself only when it resides inside the cell of another organism.

viscoelastic: A substance possessing both viscous and elastic properties.

viscosity: The thickness of a fluid; the resistance to flow of a fluid.

visual acuity: A measure of the sharpness or clarity of vision.

visual field: Peripheral vision.

vitamin: A natural compound essential to proper nutrition and regulation of metabolism found in natural foodstuffs and produced within the body.

vitreous humor: The clear, watery fluid found behind the lens of the eye.

VLDL: *See* very low-density lipoprotein.

volar: Pertaining to the palm of the hand or sole of the foot.

volar plate: The capsular ligaments on the palmer side of the hand or sole of the foot.

volition: Voluntary, the act of choosing.

Volkman's contracture: A contracture of the forearm flexors due to ischemia; a possible complication of forearm fracture.

volume: The total space occupied or displaced by an object, generally measured in cubic units.

vulvovaginitis: Inflammation of the vulva and vagina.

wart: Verruca; a rough benign growth of the skin caused by a virus.

Watson test: A special test for lunate/scaphoid subluxation. *See* Special Tests—Hand/Wrist (Appendix 17).

watt: The unit of electrical power; a measure of power equal to the power of one amp traveling across a potential difference of one volt; the unit of measure for ultrasound intensity.

wave: An oscillation with a defined frequency, duration, and amplitude.

waveform: In therapeutic modalities, the shape of the wave; examples include sine, square, triangular, asymmetrical, and twin peak.

wavelength: The distance from the beginning to the end of one complete waveform usually measured from the top of one wave to the same point on the top of the next.

weight: The force of gravity on a mass.

weightbearing exercise: Exercises that are performed under the stress of one's body weight.

well straight-leg raise: Special test of the lumbar spine for nerve root compression. *See* Special Tests—Spine (Appendix 17).

wheezing: A symptom of asthma and other respiratory distress syndromes in which a raspy or high-pitched sound is created due to the narrowing of the air passageway.

whiplash injury: A generic term for a neck sprain/strain that was caused by a sudden, forceful extension, followed by flexion similar to that which would occur in a vehicle accident when hit from behind.

white blood cell (WBC): The blood cells that are responsible for helping to prevent and fight off infection.

William's flexion exercises: Back and trunk exercises that
emphasize flexion such as pelvic tilt, single leg crunch
(knee to chest), and double leg crunch; sometimes exac-
erbate symptoms from disk injury.

within normal limits (WNL): Considered normal, often
used to describe range of motion at a joint, manual
muscle test, or other tests.

Wolff"s law: Law that states that bone forms in response to
the demands placed upon it. Bone that is not subjected
to stress will atrophy while bone that is stressed will
hypertrophy.

work: The force times the distance through which it is
applied. $w = f \times d$.

X

Xanthine: An inhaler used to treat asthma through its action to dilate the bronchioles.

xeroderma: Rough, dry skin.

x-ray: *See* radiography.

Y

yeast infection: Relating to a candidiasis infection.

Yeoman's test: A special test of the lumbar spine, hip, and/or sacroiliac joint. *See* Special Tests—SI Joint (Appendix 17).

Yergason's test: A special test of the shoulder to determine the presence of biceps tendonitis or biceps tendon subluxation. *See* Special Tests—Shoulder (Appendix 17).

yield point: Elastic limit; the point on a stress-strain curve at which further stress will cause permanent deformation.

LIST OF APPENDICES

Appendix 1

Medical Roots Terminology

Reprinted with permission from Bottomley J. *Quick Reference Dictionary for Physical Therapy.* Thorofare, NJ: SLACK Incorporated; 2000.

a-	negative prefix; eg, ametria (n is added before words beginning with a vowel)
ab-	away from; eg, abducent
abdomin-	abdomen; eg, abdominis, abdominoscopy
ac-	*see* ad-; eg, accretion
ac-	pertaining to
acet-	acid; eg, acetum vinegar, acetometer
acid-	acid; eg, acidus sour, aciduric
acou-	hear; eg, acouesthesia (also spelled acu-)
acr-	extremity, peak; eg, acromegaly
act-	drive, act; eg, reaction
actin-	ray, radius; eg, actinogenesis
acu-	hear; eg, osteoacusis
ad-	toward (d changes to c, f, g, p, s, or t before words beginning with those consonants); eg, adrenal
aden-	gland; eg, adenoma
adeno-	gland
adip-	fat; eg, adipocellular, adipose
-aemia	blood; eg, polycythaemia
aer-	air; eg, anaerobiosis
aero-	air
aesthe-	sensation; eg, aesthesioneurosis
af-	*see* ad-; eg, afferent
ag-	*see* ad-; eg, agglutinant
-agogue	leading, inducing; eg, galactagogue
-agra	catching, seizure; eg, podagra

al-	pertaining to white; eg, albocinereous
albo-	white
alg-	pain; eg, neuralgia, algesia
all-	other, different; eg, allergy
alve-	channel, cavity; eg, alveolar, alveous trough
amb-	both, on both sides; eg, ambulate
amph-	*see* amphi-, around, on both sides; eg, ampheclexis
amphi-	both, doubly (i is dropped before words beginning with a vowel); eg, amphicelous
amyl-	starch; eg, amylosynthesis
an-	pertaining to
an-	*see* ana-; eg, anagogic
ana-	up, positive (final a is dropped before words beginning with a vowel); eg, anaphoresis
andr-	man; eg, gynandroid
angi-	vessel; eg, angiemphraxis
angio-	vessel
aniso-	unequal
ankyl-	crooked, looped; eg, ankylodactylia (also spelled ancyl-)
ant-	*see* anti-; eg, antophthalmic
ante-	before; eg, anteflexion
anti-	against, counter (i is dropped before words beginning with a vowel or the word is hyphenated); eg, antipyogenic, anti-inflammatory (*see also* contra-)
antr-	cavern; eg, antrodynia
ap-	*see* ad-; eg, append
-aph-	touch; eg, dysaphia (*see also* hapt-)
apo-	away from, detached, opposed (o is dropped before words beginning with a vowel); eg, apophysis
ar-	pertaining to

arachn-	spider; eg, arachnodactyly
arch-	beginning, origin; eg, archenteron
arter(i)-	elevator, artery; eg, arteriosclerosis, periarteritis
arthr-	joint; eg, synarthrosis (*see also* articul-)
arthro-	joint
articul-	articulus joint; eg, disarticulation (*see also* arthr-)
as-	*see* ad-; eg, assimilation
-ase	enzyme
at-	*see* ad-; eg, attrition
audio-	hearing
aur-	ear; eg, aurinasal (*see also* ot-)
aut-	self; eg, autechoscope
auto-	self; eg, autoimmune
aux-	increase; eg, enterauxe
ax-	axis; eg, axofugal
axon-	axis; eg, axonometer
ba-	go, walk, stand; eg, hypnobatia
bacill-	small staff, rod; eg, actinobacillosis (*see also* bacter-)
bacter-	small staff, rod; eg, bacteriophage (*see also* bacill-)
ball-	throw; eg, ballistics (*see also* bol-)
bar-	weight; eg, pedobarometer
bi-	life; eg, aerobic
bi-	two, twice, double; eg, bipedal
bil-	bile; eg, biliary
bio-	life
blast-	bud, child, a growing thing in its early stages; eg, blastoma, zygotoblast
blep-	look; eg, hemiablepsia
blephar-	eyelid; eg, blepharoncus
bol-	ball; eg, embolism
brachi-	arm; eg, brachiocephalic
brachy-	short; eg, brachycephalic

brady-	slow; eg, bradycardia
brom-	stench; eg, podobromidrosis
bronch-	windpipe; eg, bronchoscopy
bry-	be full of life; eg, embryonic
bucc-	cheek; eg, distobuccal
cac-	bad, evil, abnormal; eg, cacodontia, arthrocace (*see also* mal-, dys-)
calc-	stone, limestone, lime; eg, calcipexy
calc-	heel; eg, calcaneotibial
calor-	heat; eg, calorimeter (*see also* therm-)
cancr-	cancer, crab; eg, cancrology (*see also* carcin-)
capit-	head; eg, decapitate (*see also* cephal-)
caps-	container; eg, encapsulation
carbo-	coal, charcoal; eg, carbohydrate, carbonuria
carcin-	crab, cancer; eg, carcinoma (*see also* cancr-)
cardi-	heart; eg, lipocardiac
cardio-	heart
cat-	*see* cata-; eg, cathode
cata-	down, negative (final a is dropped before words beginning with a vowel); eg, catabatic
caud-	tail; eg, caudate
cav-	hollow; eg, concave
cec-	blind; eg, cecopexy
-cele	tumor, hernia, cyst; eg, gastrocele
cell-	room; eg, celliferous
cen-	common; eg, cenesthesia
cent-	one hundred; eg, centimeter, centipede
cente-	puncture; eg, enterocentesis, amniocentesis
centr-	central point, center; eg, neurocentral
cephal-	relating to the head; eg, encephalitis
cept-	take, receive; eg, receptor

cer-	wax; eg, ceroplasty, ceromel
cerebr-	relating to the cerebrum; eg, cerebrospinal
cervic-	neck; eg, cervicitis, cervical
chancr-	crab, cancer; eg, chancriform
chir-	hand; eg, chiromegaly
chlor-	green; eg, achloropsia
chloro-	green
chol-	bile; eg, hepatocholangeitis
chondr-	cartilage; eg, chondromalcia
chondro-	cartilage
chord-	string, cord; eg, perichordal
chori-	protective fetal membrane; eg, endochorion
chrom-	color; eg, polychromatic
chron-	time; eg, synchronous
chy-	pour; eg, ecchymosis
-cid(e)	causing death, cut, kill; eg, infanticide, germicidal
cili-	eyelid; eg, superciliary (*see also* blephar-)
cine-	move; eg, autocinesis
-cipient	take, receive; eg, incipient
circum-	around; eg, circumferential (*see also* peri-)
-cis-	cut, kill; eg, excision
clas-	break; eg, osteoclast, cranioclast
clin-	bend, incline, make lie down; eg, clinometer
clus-	shut; eg, malocclusion
co-	*see* con-; eg, cohesion
cocc-	seed, pill; eg, gonococcus
coel-	hollow; eg, coelenteron (also spelled cel-)
col-	before l; com- before b, m, or p; cor- before r; eg, contraction
col-	pertaining to the lower intestine; eg, colic

col-	*see* con-; eg, collapse
colic-	large intestines
colon-	lower intestine; eg, colonic
colp-	hollow, vagina; eg, endocolpitis
com-	*see* con-; eg, commasculation
con-	with, together (becomes co- before vowels or h)
contra-	against, counter; eg, contraindication (*see also* anti-)
copr-	dung; eg, coproma (*see also* sterco-)
cor-	doll, little image, pupil; eg, isocoria
cor-	*see* con-; eg, corrugator
corpor-	body; eg, intracorporal (*see also* somat-)
cortic-	bark, rind; eg, corticosterone
cost-	rib; eg, intercostal (*see also* pleur-)
crani-	skull, cranium; eg, pericranium
cranio-	skull
creat-	meat, flesh; eg, creatorrhea
-crescent	grow; eg, excrescent
cret-	grow; eg, accretion
cret-	distinguish, separate off; eg, discrete
crin-	distinguish, separate off; eg, endocrinology
crur-	shin, leg; eg, brachiocrural
cry-	cold; eg, cryesthesia
crypt-	hide, conceal; eg, cryptorchism
cult-	tend, cultivate; eg, culture
cune-	wedge; eg, sphencuneiform
cut-	skin; eg, subcutaneous (*see also* derm[at]-)
cyan-	blue; eg, anthocyanin
cycl-	circle, cycle; eg, cyclophoria
cyst-	bag, bladder; eg, nephrocystitis (*see also* vesic-)
cyt-	cell; eg, plasmocytoma (*see also* cell-)
cyto	cell

dacry-	tear; eg, dacryocyst
dactyl-	finger, toe, digit; eg, hexadactylism
de-	down from; eg, decomposition
dec-	ten, indicates multiple in metric system; eg, decagram
dec-	ten, indicates fraction in metric system; eg, decimeter
deci-	tenth; eg, decibel
demi-	half; eg, demipenniform
dendr-	tree; eg, neurodendrite
dent-	tooth; eg, interdental (*see also* odont-)
dento-	teeth
derm-	skin; eg, endoderm, dermatitis (*see also* cut-)
derma-	skin
-desis	binding, stabilization
desm-	band, ligament; eg, syndesmopexy
dextr-	handedness; eg, ambidextrous
di-	two; eg, dimorphic (*see also* bi-2)
di-	*see* dia-; eg, diuresis
di-	*see* dis-; eg, divergent
dia-	through, apart, between, asunder (a is dropped before words beginning with a vowel); eg, diagnosis
didym-	twin, gemini; eg, epididymal
digit-	finger, toe; eg, digital (*see also* dactyl-)
diplo-	double; eg, diplomyelia
dips-	thirst
dis-	apart, away from, negative, absence of (s may be dropped before a word beginning with a consonant); eg, dislocation
disc-	disk; eg, discoplacenta
dors-	back; eg, ventrodorsal
drom-	course; eg, hemodromometer
-ducent	lead, conduct; eg, adducent
duct-	lead, conduct; eg, oviduct
dur-	hard, sclera; eg, induration

dynam(i)-	power; eg, dynamoneure, neurodynamic
-dynia	pain; eg, coxodynia
dys-	bad, improper, malfunction, difficult; eg, dystrophic
e-	out from; eg, emission
-eal	pertaining to
ec-	out of, on the outside; eg, eccentric
-ech-	have, hold, be; eg, synechotomy
ect-	outside; eg, ectoplasm (*see also* extra-)
ecto-	out, without, away
-ectomy	a cutting out; eg, mastectomy
ede-	swell; eg, edematous
ef-	out of; eg, efflorescent
-elc-	sore, ulcer; eg, enterelcosis (*see also* helc-)
electr-	amber; eg, electrotherapy
em-	in, on; eg, embolism, empathy, emphlysis (*see also* en-)
-em-	blood; eg, anemia (*see also* hem[at]-)
-emesis	vomiting; eg, nemesis
-emia	blood; eg, bacteremia
en-	in, on, into (n changes to m before b, p, or ph); eg, encelitis
encephal-	brain
end-	inside; eg, endangium (*see also* intra-)
endo-	within; eg, endocardium
enter-	intestine; eg, dysentery
epi-	upon, after, in addition (i is dropped before words beginning with a vowel); eg, epiglottis, epaxial
erg-	work, deed; eg, energy
erid/o-	iris (eye)
erythr-	red, rubor; eg, erythrochromia
erythro-	red
eso-	inside; eg, esophylactic (*see also* intra-, endo-)

esophag/o-	esophagus
-esthe-	perceive, feel, sensation; eg, anesthesia
eu-	good, normal, well; eg, eupepsia, eugeric
ex-	out of; eg, excretion
exo-	outside; eg, exopathic (*see also* extra-)
extra-	outside of, beyond; eg, extracellular
faci-	face; eg, brachiofaciolingual
-facient	make; eg, calefacient
-fact-	make; eg, artefact
fasci-	band; eg, fascia
febr-	fever; eg, febrile, febricide
-fect-	make; eg, defective
-ferent	bear, carry; eg, efferent, afferent
ferr-	iron; eg, ferroprotein
fibr-	fiber; eg, chondofibroma
fibro-	fiber
fil-	thread; eg, filament, filiform
fiss-	split; eg, fissure
flagell-	whip; eg, flagellation
flav-	yellow; eg, riboflavin
-flect-	bend, divert; eg, deflection
-flex-	bend, divert; eg, reflexometer, flexion
flu-	flow; eg, fluid
flux-	flow; eg, affluxion
for-	door, opening; eg, foramen, perforated
fore-	before, in front of; eg, forefront
-form	shape, form; eg, ossiform, cuniform
fract-	break; eg, fracture, refractive
front-	forehead, front; eg, nasofrontal
-fug(e)	to drive away, flee, avoid; eg, vermifuge, centrifugal
funct-	perform, serve, function; eg, functional, malfunction
fund-	pour; eg, infundibulum
fus-	pour; eg, diffusible

galact-	milk; eg, dysgalactia
gam-	marriage, reproductive union; eg, agamont
gangli-	swelling, plexus; eg, neurogangliitis
gastro-	stomach, belly; eg, gastrostomy
gelat-	freeze, congeal; eg, gelatin
gemin-	twin, double; eg, quadrigeminal
gen-	become, be produced, originate, formation; eg, genesis, cytogenic, gene
-genesis	beginning
germ-	bud, a growing thing in its early stages; eg, germinal, ovigerm
gest-	bear, carry; eg, congestion
gland-	acorn; eg, intraglandular
-glia	glue; eg, neuroglia
gloss-	relating to the tongue; eg, lingutrichoglossia
glott-	tongue, language; eg, glottic
gluc-	sweet; eg, glucose
glutin-	glue; eg, agglutination
glyco-	sugar
glyc(y)-	sweet; eg, glycemia, glycyrrhia
gnath-	jaw; eg, orthognathous
gno-	know, discern; eg, diagnosis
gon-	produce, formulate; eg, gonad, amphigony
grad-	walk, take steps; eg, retrograde
-gram	scratch, write, record; eg, cardiogram
gran-	grain, particle; eg, lipogranuloma, granulation
graph-	scratch, write, record; eg, histography
grav-	heavy; eg, multigravida
gyn(ec)-	woman, wife; eg, androgyny, gynecologic
gyr-	ring, circle; eg, gyrospasm

haem(at)-	pertaining to blood; eg, haemorrhagia, haematoxylon
hapt-	touch; eg, haptometer
hect-	one hundred, indicates multiple in metric system; eg, hectometer
helc-	sore, ulcer; eg, helcosis
hem(at)-	blood; eg, hematocyturia, hemangioma
hemi	half; eg, hemiageusia (*see also* semi-)
hemo-	blood
hen-	one; eg, henogenesis
hepat-	liver; eg, gastrohepatic
hept(a)-	seven; eg, heptatomic, heptavalent
hered-	heir; eg, heredity
hetero-	other, indicating dissimilarity; eg, heterogeneous
hex-	six, sex-, hexly-; eg, hexagram
hex-	have, hold, be; eg, cachexy
hexa-	six, sex-, hexly-; eg, hexachromic
hidr-	sweat; eg, hyperhidrosis
hist-	web, tissue; eg, histodialysis
hod-	road, path; eg, hodoneuromere
holo-	all; eg, hologenesis
homo-	common, same; eg, homomorphic
horm-	impetus, impulse; eg, hormone
hydat-	water; eg, hydatism
hydr-	pertaining to water; eg, achlorhydria
hydro-	water
hyp-	under; eg, hypaxial, hypodermic
hyper-	over, above, beyond, extreme; eg, hypertrophy
hypn-	sleep; eg, hypnotic
hypo-	under, below (o is dropped before words beginning with a vowel); eg, hypometabolism
hyster-	womb; eg, hysterectomy

-ia	condition of
-iasis	condition, pathological state; eg, hemiathriasis (*see also* -osis)
iatr-	specialty in medicine; eg, pediatrics
-ic	pertaining to
idio-	peculiar, separate, distinct; eg, idiosyncrasy
il-	negative prefix (eg, illegible); in, on (eg, illinition)
ile-	pertaining to the ileum (ile- is commonly used to refer to the portion of the intestines known as the ileum); eg, ileostomy
ili-	lower abdomen, intestines, (ili- is commonly used to refer to the flaring part of the hip bone known as the ilium); eg, iliosacral
im-	in, on (eg, immersion); negative prefix (eg, imperfection)
in-	fiber; eg, inosteatoma
in-	in, on (n changes to l, m, or r before words beginning with those consonants); eg, insertion
in-	negative prefix; eg, invalid
infra-	beneath; eg, infraorbital
insul-	island; eg, insulin
inter-	among, between; eg, intercarpal
intra-	inside; eg, intravenous
ir-	in, on (eg, irradiation); negative prefix (eg, irreducible)
irid-	rainbow, colored circle; eg, keratoiridocyclitis
is-	equal; eg, isotope
ischi-	hip, haunch; eg, ischiopubic
-ism	condition, theory; eg, hemiballism, agism
iso-	equal; eg, isotonic

-ist	specialist
-itis	inflammation; eg, neuritis
-ive	pertaining to
-ize	to treat by special method; eg, special-ize
jact-	throw; eg, jactitation
ject-	throw; eg, injection
jejun-	hungry, not partaking of food; eg, gastrojejunostomy
jug-	yoke; eg, conjugation
junct-	yoke, join; eg, conjunctiva
juxta-	near; eg, juxtaposed
kary-	nut, kernel, nucleus; eg, megakaryocyte
kerat-	horn; eg, keratolysis, keratin
kil-	one thousand, indicates multiple in metric system; eg, kilogram
kine-	move; eg, kinematics
kinesio-	movement
-kinesis	movement; eg, orthokinesis
labi-	lip; eg, gingivolabial
lact-	milk; eg, glucolactone, lactose
lal-	talk, babble; eg, glossolalia
lapar-	flank, loin, abdomen; eg, laparotomy
laryng-	windpipe; eg, laryngendoscope
lat-	ear, carry; eg, translation
later-	side; eg, bentrolateral
lent-	lentil; eg, lenticonus
lep-	take, seize; eg, cataleptic, epileptic
lepto-	small, soft; eg, leptotene
leuk-	white; eg, leukocyte (also spelled leuc-)
lien-	spleen; eg, lienocele
lig-	tie, bind; eg, ligate
lingu-	tongue; eg, sublingual

lip-	fat; eg, glycolipid
lipo-	fat
lith-	stone; eg, nephrolithotomy
litho-	stone
loc-	place; eg, locomotion
log-	speak, give an account; eg, logorrhea, embryology
-logy	study of
lumb-	loin; eg, dorsolumbar
lute-	yellow; eg, xanthluteoma
ly-	loose, dissolve; eg, keratolysis
lymph-	water; eg, hydrolymphadenosi
-lysis	setting free, disintegration; eg, glycolysis
macro-	long, large; eg, marcromyoblast
mal-	bad, abnormal; eg, malfunction
malac-	soft; eg, osteomalacia
mamm-	breast; eg, mammogram, mammary
man-	hand; eg, maniphalanx, manipulation
mani-	mental aberration; eg, kleptomania
-mania	excessive preoccupation
mast-	breast; eg, mastectomy, hypermastia
medi-	middle; eg, medial, medifrontal
mega-	great, large, indicates multiple (1 million) in metric system; eg, megacolon, megadyne
megal-	great, large; eg, cardiomegaly, acromegaly
mel-	limb, member; eg, symmelia
melan-	black; eg, melanoma, melanin
melano-	black
men-	month; eg, menopause, dysmenorrhea
mening-	membrane; eg, encephalomeningitis
ment-	mind; eg, dementia
mer-	part; eg, polymeric
mes-	middle; eg, mesoderm

meso-	middle
met-	after, beyond, accompanying; eg, met-allergy
meta-	after, beyond, accompanying (a is dropped before words beginning with a vowel); eg, metacarpal, metatarsal
-meter	measure
metr-	measure; eg, stereometry
metr-	womb; eg, endometritis
micr-	small; eg, photomicrograph
micro-	small
mill-	one thousand, indicates fraction in metric system; eg, milligram, millipede
mio-	smaller, less; eg, mionectic
miss-	send; eg, intromission
-mittent	send; eg, intermittent
mne-	remember; eg, pseudomnesia
mon-	only, sole, single; eg, monoplegia
mono-	single
morph-	form, shape; eg, morphonuclear
mot-	move; eg, vasomotor, locomotion
multi-	many; eg, multiple
my-	muscle; eg, myopathy
-myces	fungus; eg, myelomyces
myc(et)-	fungus; eg, ascomycetes, streptomycin
myel-	marrow; eg, poliomyelitis
myo-	muscle
myx-	mucus; eg, myxedema
narc-	numbness; eg, toponarcosis, narcolepsy
nas-	nose; eg, nasal
necr-	corpse, dead; eg, necrocytosis, necrosis
necro-	dead
neo-	new, young; eg, neocyte, neonate
nephr-	kidney; eg, nephron, nephric
nephro-	kidney

neur-	nerve; eg, neurology, estesioneure
neuro-	nerve and brain
nod-	knot; eg, nodosity
nom-	deal out, distribute, law, custom; eg, nominal, taxonomy
non-	nine, no; eg, nonacosane
nos-	disease; eg, nosology
nucle-	nut, kernel; eg, nucleus, nucleide
nutri-	nourish; eg, malnutrition
nyct-	night
ob-	against, toward (b changes to c before words beginning with that consonant); eg, obtuse
oc-	*see* ob-, occlude
ocul-	eye; eg, oculomotor
-od-	road, path; eg, periodic
-ode	road, path; eg, cathode
-ode	form; eg, nematode
odont-	tooth; eg, orthodontia
-odyn-	pain, distress; eg, gastrodynia
-oid	form; resembling; eg, hyoid;
-ol	oil; eg, cholesterol
-old	form, shape, resemblance; eg, scaffold
ole-	oil; eg, oleorsin
olig-	few, small; eg, oligospermia
-oma	tumor; eg, blastoma
omo-	shoulder; eg, omosternum
omphal-	navel; eg, periomphalic
onc-	bulk, mass; eg, oncology, hematoncometry
onych-	claw, nail; eg, anonychia
oo-	egg, ovum; eg, perioothecitis
oophor-	pertaining to the ovary; eg, oophorectomy
ophthalm-	eye; eg, ophthalmic
or-	mouth; eg, intraoral

orb-	circle; eg, suborbital
orchi-	testicle; eg, orchiopathy
organ-	implement, instrument; eg, organoleptic
-orrhage	excessive bleeding
-orrhagia	hemorrhage
-orrhaphy	suture
-orrhea	flow, discharge
-orrhexis	rupture
orth-	straight, right, normal; eg, orthopedics
-osis	condition, disease; eg, osteoporosis
oss-	bone; eg, osseous, ossiphone
ost(e)-	bone; eg, enostosis, osteonecrosis
-ostomy	new opening
ot-	ear; eg, parotid (*see also* aur-)
oto-	ear
-otomy	cutting; eg, osteotomy
-ous	pertaining to
ov-	egg; eg, synovia
oxy-	sharp, acid; eg, oxycephalic
pachy(n)-	thicken; eg, pachyderma, myopachynsis
pag-	fix, make fast; eg, thoracopagus
pan-	entire, all; eg, pancytosis, pandemic
par-	bear, give birth to; eg, primiparous
par-	*see* para-; eg, parepigastric
para-	beside, beyond, along side of (final a is dropped before words beginning with a vowel); eg, paramastoid
part-	bear, give birth to; eg, parturition
path-	that which one undergoes, sickness, disease; eg, pathology, psychopathic
patho-	disease
pec-	fix, make fast; eg, sympectothiene (*see also* pex-)
ped-	child; eg, pediatric, orthopedic

pell-	skin, hide; eg, pellagra
-pellent	drive; eg, repellent
pen-	need, lack; eg, erythrocytopenia
pend-	hang down; eg, appendix
-penia	deficiency
pent(a)-	five; eg, pentose, pentaploid
peps-	digest; eg, bradypepsia
pept-	digest; eg, dyspeptic
per-	through, excessive; eg, pernasal
peri-	around; eg, periphery
pet-	seek, tend toward; eg, centripetal
pex-	fix, make fast; eg, hepatopexy
-pexy	fixation
pha-	say, speak; eg, dysphasia
phac-	lentil, lens; eg, phacosclerosis (also spelled phak-)
phag-	eat; eg, lipphagic
phak-	lentil, lens; eg, phakitis
phan-	show, be seen; eg, diaphanoscopy
pharmac-	drug; eg, pharmacology
pharyng-	throat; eg, glossopharyngeal
phen-	show, be seen; eg, phosphene
pher-	bear, support; eg, periphery
phil-	like, have affinity for; eg, eosinophilia, philosophy
phleb-	vein; eg, periphlebitis, phlebotomy
phleg-	burn, inflame; eg, adenophlegmon
phlog-	burn, inflame; eg, antiphlogistic
phob-	fear, dread; eg, claustrophobia
-phobia	fear
phon-	sound; eg, echophony
phono-	voice
phor-	bear, support; eg, exophoria
phos-	light; eg, phosphorus
phot-	light; eg, photerythrous
phrag-	fence, wall off, stop up; eg, diaphragm
phrax-	fence, wall off, stop up; eg, emphraxis

phren-	mind, midriff; eg, metaphrenia, metaphrenon
phthi-	decay, waste away; eg, opthalmophthisis
phy-	beget, bring forth, produce, be by nature; eg, nosophyte, physical
phyl-	tribe, kind; eg, phylogeny
phylac-	guard; eg, prophylactic
-phylaxis	protection; eg, prophylaxis
-phyll	leaf; eg, xanthophyll
phys(a)-	blow, inflate; eg, physocele, physalis
physe-	blow, inflate; eg, emphysema
pil-	hair; eg, epilation
pituit-	phlegm; eg, pituitous
placent-	cake; eg, extraplacental
plas-	mold, shape; eg, cineplasty, plastazode
-plasty	surgical repair
platy-	broad, flat; eg, platyrrhine
pleg-	strike; eg, diplegia, paraplegia
plet-	fill; eg, depletion
pleur-	rib, side; eg, peripleural
plex-	strike; eg, apoplexy
plic-	fold; eg, complication
plur-	more; eg, plural
pne-	breathing; eg, traumatopnea
-pnea	breathing
pneum(at)-	breath, air; eg, pneumodynamics, pneumothorax
pneumo(n)-	lung; eg, pneumocentesis, pneumontomy
pod-	foot; eg, podiatry
poie-	make, produce; eg, sarcopoietic
pol-	axis of a sphere; eg, peripolar
poly-	much, many; eg, polyspermia
pont-	bridge; eg, pontocerebellar
por-	passage; eg, myelopore
por-	callus; eg, porocele

posit-	put, place; eg, deposit, repositor
post-	after, behind in time or place; eg, post-natal, postural
pre-	before in time or place; eg, prenatal, prevesical
press-	press; eg, pressure, pressoreceptive
pro-	before in time or place; eg, progamous, prolapse
proct-	anus; eg, ecteroproctia
prosop-	face; eg, prosopus
proto-	first; eg, prototype
pseud-	false; eg, pseudoparaplegia
psych-	soul, mind; eg, psychosomatic
pto-	fall; eg, nephroptosis
-ptosis	prolapse
pub-	adult; eg, puberty, ischiopubic
puber-	adult; eg, puberty
pulmo(n)-	lung; eg, cardiopulmonary, pulmolith
puls-	drive; eg, propulsion
punct-	prick, pierce; eg, puncture, punctiform
pur-	pus; eg, puration
py-	pus; eg, nephropyosis
pyel-	trough, basin, pelvis; eg, nephropyelitis
pyl-	door, orifice; eg, pylephlebitis
pyo-	pus
pyr-	fire; eg, galactopyra
quadr-	four; eg, quadraplegic, quadrigeminal
quinque-	five; eg, quinquecuspid
rachi-	spine; eg, alorachidian
radi-	ray; eg, irradiation
re-	back, again; eg, retraction
ren-	kidneys; eg, adrenal
ret-	net; eg, retothelium

retro-	backward; eg, retrodeviation, retrograde
rhag-	break, burst; eg, hemorrhagic
rhaph-	suture, stitching; eg, gastrorrhaphy
rhe-	flow, discharge; eg, disrrheal
rhex-	break, burst; eg, metrorrhexis
rhin-	nose; eg, basirhinal
rhino-	nose
-rhod	red
rot-	wheel; eg, rotator
rub(r)-	red; eg, bilirubin, rubrospinal
sacchar-	sugar; eg, saccharin
sacro-	pertaining to the sacrum; eg, sacroiliac
salping-	tube, trumpet; eg, salpingitis
sanguin-	blood; eg, sanguineous
sarc-	flesh; eg, sarcoma
schis-	split; eg, schistorachis, rachischisis
scler-	hard; eg, sclerosis, scleraderma
sclero-	hardening
scop-	look at, observe; eg, endoscope
sect-	cut; eg, sectile, resection
semi-	half; eg, semiflexion
sens-	perceive, feel; eg, sensory
sep-	rot, decay; eg, sepsis
sept-	fence, wall off, stop up; eg, septal
sept-	seven; eg, septan
ser-	whey, watery substance; eg, serum, serosynovitis
sex-	six; eg, sexdigitate
sial-	saliva; eg, polysialia
sin-	hollow, fold; eg, sinobronchitis
sit-	food; eg, parasitic
solut-	loosen, dissolve, set free; eg, dissolution
-solvent	loosen, dissolve; eg, dissolvent

somat-	body; eg, somatic, psychosomatic
-some	body; eg, dictyosome
spas-	draw, pull; eg, spasm, spastic
spectr-	appearance, what is seen; eg, spectrum, microspectroscope
sperm(at)-	seed; eg, spermacrasia, spermatozoon
spers-	scatter; eg, dispersion
sphen-	wedge; eg, sphenoid
spher-	ball; eg, hemisphere
sphygm-	pulsation; eg, sphygmomanometer
spin-	spine; eg, cerebrospinal
spirat-	breathe; eg, inspiratory
splanchn-	entrails, vicera; eg, neurosplanchnic
splen-	spleen; eg, splenomegaly
spor-	seed; eg, sporophyte, sygospore
squam-	scale; eg, squamus, desquamation
sta-	make stand, stop; eg, genesistasis
stal-	send; eg, peristalsis (*see also* stol-)
staphyl-	bunch of grapes, uvula; eg, staphylococcus, staphylectomy
-stasis	stopping, controlling
stear-	fat; eg, stearodermia
steat-	fat; eg, steatopygous
sten-	narrow, compressed; eg, stenocardia
ster-	solid; eg, cholesterol
sterc-	dung; eg, stercoporphyrin
sthen-	strength; eg, asthenia
stol-	send; eg, diastole
stom(at)-	mouth, orifice; eg, anastomosis, stomatogastric
strep(h)-	twist; eg, strephosymbolia, streptomycin (*see also* stroph-)
strict-	draw tight, compress, cause pain; eg, constriction
-stringent	draw tight, compress, cause pain; eg, astringent
stroph-	twist; eg, astrophic (*see also* strep[h]-)

struct-	pile up (against); eg, obstruction
sub-	under, below (b changes to f or p before words beginning with those consonants); eg, sublumbar
suf-	*see* sub-; eg, suffusion
sup-	*see* sub-; eg, suppository
super-	above, beyond, extreme; eg, supermobility
supra-	above, beyond
sy-	*see* syn-; eg, systole
syl-	*see* syn-; eg, syllepsiology
sym-	*see* syn-; eg, symbiosis, symmetry, sympathetic, symphysis
syn-	with, together (n dropped before s; changes to l before l; and changes to m before b, m, p, and ph); eg, myosynizesis
ta-	stretch, put under pressure; eg, ectasis
tac-	order, arrange; eg, atactic
tachy-	over
tact-	touch; eg, contact
tax-	order, arrange; eg, ataxia, taxotomy
tect-	cover; eg, protective
teg-	cover; eg, integument
tel-	end; eg, telosynapsis
tele-	at a distance; eg, teleceptor, telescope
tempor-	time, timely or fatal spot, temple; eg, temporomalar
ten(ont)-	tight stretched band; eg, tenodynia, tenonitis, tenontagra
tens-	stretch; eg, extensor
test-	pertaining to the testicle; eg, testitis
tetra-	four; eg, tetragenous
the-	put, place; eg, synthesis
thec-	repository, case; eg, thecostegnosis
thel-	teat, nipple; eg, thelerethism

thera-	therapy
therap-	treatment; eg, hydrotherapy
therm-	heat; eg, diathermy
thermo-	heat
thi-	sulfur; eg, thiogenic
thorac/o-	thorax (chest); eg, thoracoplasty
thromb-	lump, clot; eg, thrombophlebitis, thrombopenia
thym-	spirit; eg, dysthymia
thyr-	shield, shaped like a door; eg, thyroid
tme-	cut; eg, axonotmesis
toc-	childbirth; eg, dystocia
tom-	cut; eg, appendenctomy
ton-	stretch, put under pressure; eg, tonus, peritoneum
top-	place; eg, topesthesia
tors-	twist; eg, extorsion
tox-	arrow poison, poison; eg, toxemia
trache-	windpipe; eg, tracheotomy
trachel-	neck; eg, tracheloplexy
tract-	draw, drag; eg, protraction
trans-	across; eg, transport
traumat-	wound; eg, traumatic
tri-	three; eg, trigonad
trich-	hair; eg, trichoid
trip-	rub; eg, entripsis
trop-	turn, react; eg, sitotropism
troph-	nurture, relating to nourishment; eg, atrophy
-trophy	nutrition, growth
tuber-	swelling, node; eg, tubercle, tuberculosis
tympan/o-	eardrum
typ-	type; eg, atypical
typh-	for, stupor; eg, adenotyphus
typhl-	blind; eg, typhlectasis

uni-	one; eg, unioval
ur-	urine; eg, polyuria
uro-	urine
vacc-	cow; eg, vaccine
vagin-	sheath; eg, invaginated
vas-	vessel; eg, vascular
ven/o-	vein
ventro-	abdomen, in front of; eg, ventrolateral, ventrose
vers-	turn; eg, inversion
vert-	turn; eg, diverticulum
vesic-	bladder; eg, vesicovaginal
vit-	life; eg, devitalize
vuls-	pull, twitch; eg, convulsion
xanth-	yellow, blond; eg, xanthophyll
xantho-	yellow
-yl-	substance; eg, cacodyl
zo-	life, animal; eg, microzoaria
zyg-	yoke, union; eg, zygote, zygodactyly
zym-	ferment; eg, enzyme

APPENDIX 2

Acronyms and Abbreviations

(A): assisted
A: assessment, anterior, accommodation
A, Ath: athlete
AAROM: active assistive range of motion
ABD: abduction
AC: acromioclavicular
ac: before meals
ACE: angiotensin converting enzyme
ACL: anterior cruciate ligament
ADA: American Dental Association, American Diabetes Association, American Disabilities Act
ADD: adduction or attention deficit disorder
ADL: activities of daily living
ad lib: as desired
adm: admission
AE: above elbow
AED: automatic external defibrillator
AFO: ankle foot orthosis
AIDS: acquired immunodeficiency syndrome
AIIS: anterior inferior iliac spine
AK: above the knee
ALS: amyotrophic lateral sclerosis
am: morning
AMA: against medical advice
AMA: American Medical Association
Ant: anterior
AP: anterior-posterior
ARNP: Advanced registered nurse practitioner
AROM: active range of motion
ART: active resistive training

ASA: aspirin
ASAP: as soon as possible
ASHD: arterial sclerotic heart disease
ASIS: anterior superior iliac spine
assist: assistance
ATC: athletic trainer, certified
ATC-L: athletic trainer certified and licensed
ATH: athlete

(B): bilateral
B: both
BE: below elbow
BID: twice daily
bilat: bilateral
BK: below the knee
bm: body mechanics
BM: bowel movement
BMI: body mass index
BP: blood pressure
BPM: beats per minute
BS: blood sugar

C: centrigrade
Ca: carcinoma cancer
CAAHEP: Commission on Accreditation of Allied
Health Education Programs
CABG: coronary artery bypass graft
CAD: coronary artery disease
Cal: calories
caps: capsules
CBC: complete blood count
CBR: complete bedrest
CC, C/C: chief complaint
cc: cubic centimeter
CD: cardiovascular disease
CDC: Centers for Disease Control and Prevention
CEU: continuing education units

CHF: congestive heart failure
CHI: closed head injury
CIE: clinical instructor educator
cm: centimeter
CNS: central nervous system
c/o: complained of, complains of
COG: center of gravity
COLD: chronic obstructive lung disease
cont: continue
CO$_2$: carbon dioxide
COP: center of pressure
COPD: chronic obstructive pulmonary disease
CP: cerebral palsy, chest pain, cold pack
CPM: continuous passive motion
CPR: cardiopulmonary resuscitation
CPU: central processing unit, computer processing unit
C & S: culture and sensitivity
CSCS: certified strength and conditioning specialist
CSF: cerebrospinal fluid
CV: cardiovascular
CVA: cerebrovascular accident
CWI: crutch walking instructions
CWP: cold whirlpool
Cysto: cystoscopic examination

da or DAW: dispense as written
d/c: discontinued or discharged
Dep: dependent
Dept: department
Derm: dermatology
DHHS: Department of Health and Human Services
DIP: distal interphalangeal joint
DJP: degenerative joint pain
DM: diabetes mellitus
DNR: do not resuscitate
DO: doctor of osteopathy
DOB: date of birth

DTR: deep tendon reflex
DVT: deep vein thrombosis
Dx: diagnosis

EAP: emergency action plan
ECF: extended care facility
ECG, EKG: electrocardiogram
EEG: electroencephalogram
EENT: ear, eye, nose, throat
EIA: exercise-induced asthma
EMG: electromyelogram
EMS: emergency medical services
ENT: ear, nose, throat
ER, E.R.: emergency room
EVAL: evaluation
EX: exercise
EXT: extension

F-: fair (40%)
F+: fair (60%)
F: fair (50%)
F/b: followed by
FBS: fasting blood sugar
FH: family history
FLEX: flexion
ft: foot, feet (the measurement, not the body part)
FUO: fever, unknown origin
FWB: full weightbearing
FX: fracture
FY: fiscal year

G: good (muscle strength, balance)
g or gm: gram
GB: gallbladder
GI: gastrointestinal
GTO: golgi tendon organ
GYN: gynecology

HA, H/A: headache
Hb, Hgb: hemoglobin
HBV: hepatitis B virus
Hct: height
HCVD: hypertensive cardiovascular disease
HEENT: head, ear, eye, nose, throat
H & H, H/H: hematocrit and hemoglobin
HI: head injury
HNP: herniated nucleus pulposus
HOB: head of bed
H & P: history and physical
HP: hot pack
HR: heart rate
Hr: hour
hs: at bedtime
Ht: hematocrit
Htn: hypertension
Hx, hx: history
Hz: hertz

IB: ice bag
ICU: intensive care unit
Ila: inferiolateral angle (of the sacrum)
IM: intramuscular
IMP: impression
in: inches
Indep: independent
Inj: injury
I & O: intake and output
IP: interphalangeal
IV: intravenous

JAT: *Journal of Athletic Training*
J Orthop Sports Phys Ther: *Journal of Orthopedic and
Sports Physical Therapy*

JRC-AT: Joint Review Committee on Athletic Training
JSR: *Journal of Sport Rehabilitation*

kcal: kilocalories
kg: kilogram
KJ: knee jerk
KUB: kidney, ureter, bladder

(L): left
L: liter
Lat: lateral
LATC: licensed athletic trainer, certified
lb: pound
LBP: low back pain
LE: lower extremity
LLE: left lower extremity
LLQ: left lower quadrant
LMN: lower motor neuron
LOC: loss of consciousness
LP: lumbar puncture
LPN: licensed practical nurse
LPT: licensed physical therapist
LRP: long-range plan
LUE: left upper extremity

M: male
m: meter
ma: milliamperes
Max: maximum
MBD: minimal brain damage
MBI: mild brain injury
MC: metacarpal
MCP: metacarpophalangeal
MD: medical doctor; doctor of medicine
MED: minimum effective dose
Meds: medications
MFR: myofacial release

MFT: muscle function test
mg: milligram
MHI: mild head injury
MI: myocardial infarction
min: minutes
mL: milliliter
mm: millimeter
MMT: manual muscle test
mo: month
Mod: moderate
MRI: magnetic resonance imaging
MS: multiple sclerosis
MTP: metatarsophalangeal

N: normal (muscle strength)
NATA: National Athletic Trainers' Association
NATA-BOC: NATA Board of Certification
NDT: neurodevelopmental treatment
Neg: negative
N.H.: nursing home
NIH: National Institutes of Health
NKA: no known allergy
NMES: neuromuscular electrical stimulator
noc: night, at night
NOCSAE: National Operating Committee on
     Standards for Athletic Equipment
NPO: nothing by mouth
NSAID: nonsteroidal anti-inflammatory drugs
NSR: normal sinus rhythm
NT: not tested
NWB: nonweightbearing

O: objective
OA: osteoarthritis
OBS: organic brain syndrome, observation
OD: once daily
OP: outpatient

OR: operating room
ORIF: open reduction, internal fixation
OT: occupational therapist, occupational therapy
OTC: over the counter
oz: ounce

(p): pain
P: plan (treatment plan), poor (muscle strength, balance)
P.A.: physician's assistant
PA: posterior/anterior
PARA: paraplegia
p.c., pc: after meals
PE: physical examination
PEARLS: pupils, equal and reactive to light simultaneously
per: by or through
per os, PO: by mouth
PERRLA: pupils equal, round, reactive to light and accommodations
PH: past history
PID: pelvic inflammatory disease
PIIS: posterior inferior illiac spine
PIP: proximal interphalangeal joint
PMH: previous medical history
PNF: proprioceptive neuromuscular facilitation
PNI: peripheral nerve injury
POMR: problem-oriented medical record
pos: positive
poss: possible
post: after or behind
Postop: after surgery (operation)
PRE: progressive resistive exercise
Preop: before surgery (operation)
prn: whenever necessary
PROM: passive range of motion
PSIS: posterior superior iliac spine

PT: physical therapy, physical therapist
PT, pt: patient
PTA: physical therapist assistant, prior to admission
PTB: patella tendon bearing
PVD: peripheral vascular disease
PWB: partial weightbearing

q: every
q2h: every 2 hours
q3h: every 3 hours
q4h: every 4 hours
qd: once a day
qh: every hour
qid: four times a day
qn: every night
qt.: quart

(R): right
RA: rheumatoid arthritis
RBC: red blood count
R.D.: registered dietician
re: regarding
Rehab: rehabilitation
resp: respiratory, respiration
RICE: rest, ice, compression, elevation
RICER: rest, ice, compression, elevation, rehabilitation
RLE: right lower extremity
RM: repetition maximum
RN: registered nurse
RO: rule out
ROM: range of motion
ROS: review of systems
RPE: rating of perceived exertion
RPT: registered physical therapist
RROM: resistive range of motion
R.T.: respiratory therapist
RUE: right upper extremity
Rx: treatment prescription, therapy

SACH: solid ankle cushion heel
SATA: Student Athletic Trainers' Association
SCFE: slipped capital femoral epiphysis
SC joint: sternoclavicular joint
sec: seconds
SED: suberythemal dose
SIDS: sudden infant death syndrome
Sig: directions for use, give as follows, let it be labeled
SI(J): sacroiliac (joint)
SLE: systemic lupus erythematosus
SLR: straight leg raise
SNF: skilled nursing facility
SOAP: subjective, objective, assessment, plan
s/p: status post
spec: specimen
S & S: signs and symptoms
ST: soft tissue
Stat: immediately, at once
STD: sexually transmitted disease
STM: short-term memory
Sx: symptoms

T: trace (muscle strength)
tab: tablet
TB: tuberculosis
TBI: traumatic brain injury
tbsp, T.: tablespoon
TENS: transcutaneous electrical nerve stimulation
THR: total hip replacement
TIA: transient ischemic attack
TID: three times daily
TKR: total knee replacement
TM(J): temporomandibular (joint)
TNR: tonic neck reflex (also ATNR, STNR)
t.o.: telephone order

TOS: thoracic outlet syndrome
tsp, t.: teaspoon
TTP: tender to palpation
TUR: transurethral resection
Tx: treatment

μa: microamperes
UA: urine analysis
UE: upper extremity
UMN: upper motor neuron
Un: unable
URI: upper respiratory infection
US: ultrasound
ut dict.: as directed
UTI: urinary tract infection

VD: venereal disease
VO: verbal orders (eg, v.o. Dr. Smith/your signature)
Vol: volume
VS: vital signs

WBC: white blood cell count
w/c: wheelchair
W/cm^2: watts per square centimeter
Wk: week
WNL: within normal limits
wt.: weight
WWP: warm whirlpool

x: number of times performed

yd.: yard
y/o: years old
yr.: year

APPENDIX 3

Symbols

Reprinted with permission from Jacobs K. *Quick Reference Dictionary for Occupational Therapy.* 2nd ed. Thorofare, NJ: SLACK Incorporated; 1999.

↑	increase
↓	decrease
→	to follow
↔	to and from
1°	primary/first degree
2°	secondary/due to/second degree
3°	tertiary/third degree
@	at
α	alpha
β	beta
Δ	delta, change
n	total sample size
N	total population size
μ	micron (former term for micrometer)
π	pi, 3.1416, ratio of circumference of a circle to its diameter
√	root, square root, radical
+	plus, excess, positive
−	minus, deficiency, negative
±	plus or minus, indefinite
~	approximately
≈	approximately equal
=	equals
>	greater than
<	less than
≥	greater than or equal to
≤	less than or equal to
Σ	sum
:	ratio, "is to"
::	equality between ratios, "as"
∴	therefore

$\overline{c}$	with
$\overline{s}$	without
#	number, pound
/	per
♂	male
♀	female
✓	flexion
/	extension
↻	rotation
▼	depression, downward, caudal
▲	elevation, upward, cephalic
◄►	outward, expand

APPENDIX 4

Anatomical Terms of Orientation and Direction

anterior: front, ventral
anteroposterior: front to back
caudal: toward the tail (or feet)
cephalad: toward the head
cranial: relating to the head
decubitus: lying down
deep: underneath, further from the surface
distal: further from the beginning, further from the trunk
dorsal: back, posterior
horizontal: parallel to the floor, perpendicular to a vertical line
inferior: below, lower than
lateral: toward the side of the body
medial: toward the midline of the body
posterior: back, dorsal
posteroanterior: from back to front
pronation: internal rotation of the forearm so as to place the palm down
prone: with the front or ventral surface down, lying face down
proximal: closer toward the beginning, closer to the trunk
recumbent: lying down
sagittal: A vertical plane passing through the body from front to back. The midsagittal plane divides the body into left and right halves
superficial: on top, near the surface, shallow
superior: above
supination: external rotation of the forearm so as to place the palm up

supine: with the back or dorsal surface downward, lying face up

transverse: a horizontal plane (parallel to the ground) passing through the body

ventral: front, anterior

vertical: upright, perpendicular to horizontal

APPENDIX 5

Muscles—Origin, Insertion, Action

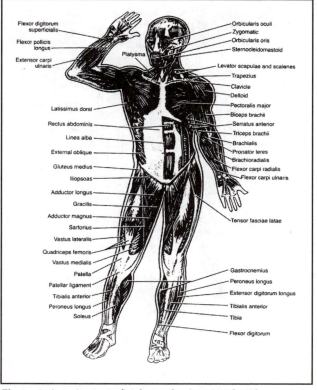

Figure 1. Anterior superficial muscles (reprinted with permission from Leonard P. *Quick and Easy Terminology.* 2nd ed. Philadelphia, Pa: WB Saunders; 1995).

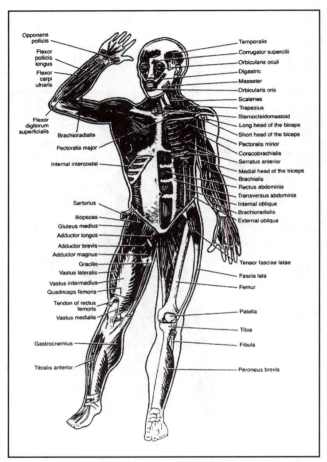

Figure 2. Anterior deep muscles (reprinted with permission from Leonard P. *Quick and Easy Terminology.* 2nd ed. Philadelphia, Pa: WB Saunders; 1995).

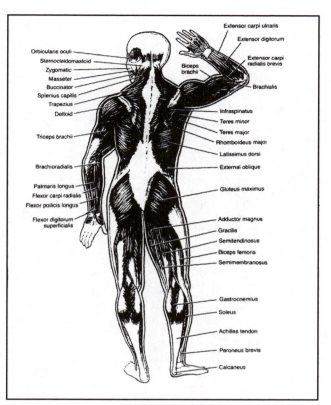

Figure 3. Posterior superficial muscles (reprinted with permission from Leonard P. *Quick and Easy Terminology*. 2nd ed. Philadelphia, Pa: WB Saunders; 1995).

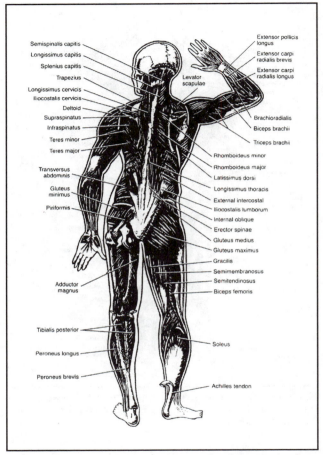

Figure 4. Posterior deep muscles (reprinted with permission from Leonard, P. *Quick and Easy Terminology*. 2nd ed. Philadelphia, Pa: WB Saunders; 1995).

MUSCLES: ORIGIN/INSERTION/ACTION—INNERVATION—BLOOD SUPPLY*

Muscle	Origin	Insertion	Action	Nerve	Artery
Neck					
Sternocleido-mastoid (SCM)	Med or sternal head cranial part of ventral surface of manubrium; lat or clavicular head—sup border & ant surface of med 1/3 clavicle	Lat surface mastoid process & lat 1/2 sup nuchal line of occipital bone	↻ opp side lat ✓ same side ✓ forward	Spinal accessory n. C2 & C3 ant rami	Subclavian a.
Platysma	Fascia covering sup part of pectoralis major & deltoid	Some fibers into bone below oblique line, others into skin	Draws lip inf & post	Cervical branch of facial n.	Subclavian a. (branch)
Suprahyoid group					
Digastricus	Post belly: mastoid notch of temporal bone; Ant belly: a depression on inner side of inf border of mandible	Post belly: hyoid bone by fibrous loop; Ant belly: same as post belly	▲ hyoid bone Post: draws backwards Ant: draws forward	Post: facial n. Ant: mylohyoid n.	Lingual a.
Stylohyoideus	Post & lat surface of styloid process	Body of hyoid bone	Draws hyoid sup & post	Facial n. (branch)	Lingual a.

Note: Please refer to key on page 235.

Muscle	Origin	Insertion	Action	Nerve	Artery
Neck					
Mylohyoideus	Whole length of mylohyoid line of mandible	Body of hyoid bone	▲ hyoid & tongue	Mylohyoid n.	Lingual a.
Geniohyoideus	Inf mental spine on inner surface of symphysis menti	Ant surface of hyoid	Draws hyoid & tongue ant	1st cervical n. (through hypoglossal n.)	Lingual a.
Infrahyoid Group					
Sternohyoideus	Post surface of med end of clavicle, post sterno-clav lig & sup & post part of manubrium sterni	Inf border of hyoid bone	Draws hyoid inferiorly	Branch of ansa cervicalis (1st three cervical nerves)	Lingual a. Subclavian a.
Sternothyroideus	Dorsal surface of manubrium sterni (caudal of origin of sternohyoideus)	Oblique line on lamina of thyroid cartilage	Draws thyroid caudally	Branch of ansa cervicalis (1st three cervical nerves)	Lingual a. Subclavian a.
Thyrohyoideus	Oblique line on lamina of thyroid cartilage	Inf border of greater cornu of hyoid bone	Draws hyoid inferiorly Draws thyroid cartilage sup	1st & 2nd cervical n.	Lingual a. Subclavian a.
Omohyoideus	Cranial border of scapula (near or crossing scapular notch)	Caudal border of hyoid bone	Draws hyoid caudally	Branch of ansa cervicalis (1st three cervical nerves)	Subclavian a.

Muscle	Origin	Insertion	Action	Nerve	Artery
Neck					
Longus Colli	Vertical: ant surface of C5, C6, C7, T1, T2 & T3; Sup: ant tubercles of transverse processes C3, C4, C5; Inf: ant surface of T2 & T3	Vertical: ant surface of C2, C3, C4; Sup: narrow tendon into tubercle on ant arch of atlas; Inf: ant tubercles of transverse processes C5 & C6	✓neck, ↻ neck (min)	Branches of 2nd to 7th cervical nerves	Subclavian a. (thyrocervical)
Longus Capitus	Four tendinous slips from ant tubercles of transverse processes C3, C4, C5 & C6	Inf surface of the basilar part of occipital bone	Head ✓	Branches from 1st, 2nd, & 3rd cervical nerves	Subclavian a.
Rectus Capitus Anterior	Ant surface of lat mass of the atlas & from root of its transverse process	Inf surface of basilar part of occipital bone	Head ✓	Branch of 1st & 2nd cervical nerves	Subclavian a.
Rectus Capitus Lateralis	Sup surface of transverse process of atlas	Inf surface of jugular process of occipital bone	Lat ✓ head	Branch of 1st & 2nd cervical nerves	Subclavian a.
Scalenus Anterior	Ant tubercles of transverse processes of C3, C4, C5 & C6	Scalene tubercle on inner border of 1st rib & ridge on cranial surface of rib	▲1st rib, ✓head, ↻ head	Branches of lower cervical nerves	Subclavian a. (thyrocervical)

Muscle	Origin	Insertion	Action	Nerve	Artery
Neck					
Scalenus Medius	Post tubercles of transverse processes of C2, C3, C4, C5, C6 & C7	Cranial surface of 1st rib between tubercle & subclavian groove	▲ 1st rib ↙ head ↻ head	Branches from cervical nerves	Subclavian a. (thyrocervical)
Scalenus Posterior	Post tubercles of transverse processes of C5, C6 & C7	Outer surface of 2nd rib (deep to serratus anterior)	▲ 2nd rib ↙ head ↻ head	Ventral primary branches C5, C6 & C7	Subclavian a.
Back/Neck					
Serratus Posterior Superior	Caudal part of ligamentum nuchae, spinous processes C7, T1, T2 & T3; supraspinal ligament	Four digitations— cranial borders of ribs 2, 3, 4 & 5	Respiratory ▲ ribs	Ventral rami T1-T4	Subclavian a.
Serratus Posterior Inferior	Spinous processes T11, T12, L1, L2 & L3; supraspinal ligament	Four digitations into inf borders last 4 ribs (a little beyond their angles)	Respiratory Draws ribs ◂▸ & ▾	Ventral rami T9-T12	Subclavian a.
Splenius Capitis Cervicis	Caudal ½ ligamentum nuchae & spinous processes C7, T1, T2, T3 & sometimes T4	Occipital bone just inf to lat 1/3 of sup nuchal line; into mastoid process of temporal bone	/ head&neck lat ↙ same side ↻ same side	Lat branches dorsal primary cervical nerves	Subclavian a. (branches)

Muscle	Origin	Insertion	Action	Nerve	Artery
Back/Neck					
Spinalis Capitis	Usually inseparable from semispinalis capitis	Usually inseparable from semispinalis capitis	/ spine	Branch dorsal primary spinal nerves	Thoracic aorta (branch)
Semispinalis Capitis	Tips of transverse processes C7, T1, T2, T3, T4, T5, T6 & sometimes T7	Between sup & inf nuchal lines of occipital bone	/ head & neck ↻ opp side	Dorsal rami	Subclavian a. (branches)
Longissimus Capitis	Transverse processes T4 & T5 and cervicis & articular processes C4 C5, C6 & C7	Post margin of mastoid process (deep to splenius capitis & SCM)	/ head ↻ same side ↙ same side	Dorsal primary mid & lower cervical n(s).	Subclavian a. (branches)
Obliquus Capitis Inferior	Arises from apex of spinous process of axis	Inf & dorsal transverse process of atlas	↻ same side	Branch dorsal primary division suboccipital n.	Subclavian a. (branch)
Obliquus Capitis Superior	Tendinous fibers from sup surface transverse process of atlas	Occipital bone between sup & inf nucal lines (lat to semispinalis capitis)	/ head	Branch dorsal primary division suboccipital n.	Subclavian a. (branch)
Rectus Capitis Posterior Major	Spinous process of the axis	Lat part of inf nuchal line of occipital bone and surface immediately inf	/ head ↻ same side	Branch dorsal primary division suboccipital n.	Subclavian a. (branch)

Muscle	Origin	Insertion	Action	Nerve	Artery
Back/Neck					
Rectus Capitis Posterior Minor	Tendon from tubercle on post arch of atlas	Med part of the inf nuchal line of occipital bone & surface between it & foramen magnum	/ head	Branch dorsal primary division suboccipital n.	Subclavian a. (branch)
Longissimus Cervicis	Long thin tendons from apex transverse processes upper 4 or 5 thoracic vertebrae	Post tubercles of transverse processes of C2-C6	/ spine, lat ✓, ▼ ribs	Dorsal primary branch spinal nerves	Thoracic aorta (branches)
Iliocostalis Cervicis	Angles of the 3rd, 4th, 5th & 6th ribs	Post tubercles of transverse processes of C4, C5 & C6	/ spine, lat ✓, ▼ ribs	Dorsal primary branch spinal nerves	Thoracic aorta (branches)
Spinalis Cervicis	Caudal part of ligamentum nuchae, spinous process C7; sometimes T1 & T2	Spinous processes of axis; sometimes spinous process C1 & C2	/ spine	Dorsal primary branch spinal nerves	Thoracic aorta (branch)
Semispinalis Cervicis	Transverse processes of 1st five or six thoracic vertebrae	Cervical spinous processes from axis to C5	/ spine, ↻ opp side	Dorsal primary branch spinal nerves	Thoracic aorta (branch)

Muscle	Origin	Insertion	Action	Nerve	Artery
Back					
Longissimus Thoracis	Arising from erector spinae & post surfaces transverse & accessory processes of lumbar vertebrae & ant layer lumbocostal aponeurosis	Transverse processes of all thoracic vertebrae and lower 9 or 10 ribs between tubercles and angles	/ spine lat ✓ ▼ ribs	Dorsal primary branch spinal nerves	Thoracic aorta (branch)
Iliocostalis Thoracis	Flattened tendons from upper borders of angles of lower 6 ribs (med to iliocostalis lumborum)	Cranial borders of angles of 1st 6 ribs and into dorsum of transverse process C7	/ spine lat ✓ ▼ ribs	Dorsal primary branch spinal nerves	Thoracic aorta (branch)
Spinalis Thoracis	Med continuation of sacrospinalis. Arises from spinous processes of T11, T12, L1 & L2	Spinous processes of upper thoracic vertebrae	/ spine	Dorsal primary branch spinal nerves	Thoracic aorta (branch)
Semispinalis Thoracis	Transverse processes of T6-T10	Spinous processes of C6, C7, T1, T2, T3 & T4	/ spine ↻ opp side	Dorsal primary branch spinal nerves	Thoracic aorta (branch)
Iliocostalis Lumborum	Flattened tendons from upper portion of erector	Inf borders of angles of last 6 or 7 ribs	/ spine lat ✓ ▼ ribs	Dorsal primary branch spinal nerves	Thoracic aorta (branch)

Muscle	Origin	Insertion	Action	Nerve	Artery
Back					
Sacrospinalis (Erector Spinae)	Arises from broad tendon attached to mid crest of sacrum; spinous processes T11-T12 & lumbar vertebrae; supraspinal ligament to lip of iliac crests & lat crest of sacrum	Splits into longissimus, iliocostalis, spinalis, & semispinalis muscles (see respective muscles)	/ spine ↺ spine ▼ ribs lat ✓	Spinal nerves	Thoracic aorta
Multifidus	Spinous processes of each vertebra from sacrum to axis; arises from back of sacrum from aponeurosis of sacrospinalis, from med surface of post sup iliac spine & post sacroiliac ligaments	Each ascends obliquely crossing over 2-4 vertebrae and inserted into spinous process of vertebra from last lumbar to axis	/ spine ↺ opp side	Branches of dorsal primary spinal nerves	Thoracic aorta
Rotatores	Transverse process of one vertebra & insert at base of spinous process of vertebra above from the sacrum to the axis	*Rotatores longi* cross one vertebra in their oblique course. *Rotatores breves* insert in next succeeding vertebra & run horizontal	/ spine ↺ opp side	Branches of dorsal primary spinal nerves	Thoracic aorta

Muscle	Origin	Insertion	Action	Nerve	Artery
Back					
Quadratus Lumborum	Sup borders of the transverse processes L2-L5	Inf border of last rib & transverse process L1-L4	▼ last rib lat ✓	12th thoracic n. 1st lumbar n.	Iliac circumflex
Shoulder Girdle					
Trapezius	Ext occipital protuberance; med 1/3 sup nuchal line; spinous process C7, T1-T12	Post border of lat 3rd clavicle; med margin acromion; spine of the scapula	▲ &/ shoulder Abd same side ↻ opp side Retraction ▲ ↻ glen fossa ▲ glen fossa	Spinal accessory n. C3 & C4 spinal nerves	Suprascapular
Levator Scapulae	Transverse processes C1-C4	Med border scapula between sup angle & spine	Elevation Protraction / cervical spine nerves Abd same side ↻ same side	Dorsal scapular n. C3 & C4 spinal nerves	Superficial cervical a. Transverse cervical a.
Romboideus Minor	Spinous process of C7 & T1	Med border scapula at level of the spine	Elevation Retraction ▼ ↻ glen fossa	Dorsal scapular n.	Descending scapular a.
Romboideus Major	Spinous process of T2-T5	Med border scapula between spine & inf angle	Elevation Retraction ▼ ↻ glen fossa	Dorsal scapular n.	Descending scapular a.

Muscle	Origin	Insertion	Action	Nerve	Artery
Shoulder Girdle					
Latissimus Dorsi	Lumbar aponeurosis; spinous processes of T6-T12, L1-L5 & sacral vertebrae	Distal part of intertubercular groove of humerus	/ shoulder Abd shoulder Med ↻ Elevation Retraction	Thoracodorsal n. C6-C8 spinal nerves	Subscapular a.
Pectoralis Major	Ant surface sternal 1/2 clavicle; ventral surface sternum; aponeurosis of obliquus externus abdominis	Crest of greater tubercle of humerus	↙ shoulder Add shoulder Med ↻ Protract; ▲▼	Med & lat pectoral n. C5-C8 spinal nerves 1st thoracic n.	Thoraco-acromial a.
Pectoralis Minor	Ext surfaces of ribs 3, 4 & 5 near their cartilages	Caracoid process of scapula	Protraction Depression ▼ ↻ glen fossa	Med pectoral n.	Thoraco-acromial a.
Subclavius	1st rib & its cartilage near their junction	Inf aspect of clavicle in the mid 3rd	Protraction Depression	Branch from brachial plexus (sup trunk)	Thoraco-acromial a.
Serratus Anterior	Ext surfaces of ribs 1-9	Ant aspect of med border of scapula from sup to inf angle	Protraction Depression ▲ ↻ glen fossa	Long thoracic n.	Lat thoracic a.
Subscapularis	Mid 2/3 subscapular fossa; inf 2/3 groove on axillary	Lesser tubercle of humerus	Med ↻ ↙ & / Abd & add	Subscapular n.	Circumflex scapular a.

Muscle	Origin	Insertion	Action	Nerve	Artery
Shoulder Girdle					
Supraspinatus	Mid 2/3 supraspinatous fossa	Sub impression of greater tubercle of humerus	Abd / Lat ⟳ (weak) / ⟲ (weak)	Suprascapular n.	Suprascapular a.
Infraspinatus	Med 2/3 infraspinatus fossa	Mid impression of greater tubercle of humerus	Lat ⟳ / Abd & add	Suprascapular n.	Suprascapular a.
Teres Minor	Dorsal surface of axillary border of scapula	Inf impression of greater tubercle of humerus distal to inf impression	Lat ⟳ / Add	Branch of axillary n.	Post humeral circumflex a.
Teres Major	Oval area on dorsal surface of inf angle of scapula	Crest of lesser tubercle of humerus	Add / shoulder / Med ⟳	Lower subscapular n.	Circumflex scapular a.
Deltoideus	Ant border & sup surface of lat 3rd of clavicle; lat margin & sup surface of acromium; inf lip post border scapular spine	Deltoid prominence on mid of lat body of humerus	Abd shoulder / ⟲ shoulder / shoulder / Med & lat ⟳	Axillary n. from brachial plexus	Post humeral circumflex a.
Shoulder/Elbow					
Triceps Brachii	Long head: infraglenoid tuberosity of scapula;	Post proximal surface of olecranon	/ elbow / shoulder	Branches radial n.	Profunda brachii a.

Muscle	Origin	Insertion	Action	Nerve	Artery
Shoulder/Elbow					
	Lat head: post surface of humerus; Med head: post surface of humerus distal to radial groove		Add shoulder		Inf ulnar collateral a.
Brachialis	Distal 1/2 of ant-aspect of humerus	Tuberosity of ulna; rough depression on ant surface of coronoid process	✓elbow	Musculo-cutaneous n. Radial & med n.	Brachial a.
Biceps Brachii	Short head: apex of coracoid process; Long head: supraglenoid tuberosity at sup margin of glenoid	Rough post portion tuberosity of radius	✓ shoulder ✓ elbow Supination	Musculo-cutaneous n.	Brachial a.
Coracobrachialis	Apex of coracoid process	Impression at med surface & border of humerus	✓ shoulder Add shoulder	Musculo-cutaneous n.	Brachial a.
Forearm/Wrist					
Pronator Teres	Humeral head: proxi-mal to med epicondyle of humerus; Ulnar head: med side of coronoid process of ulna	Rough impression at mid of lat surface of radius	Pronation	Median n.	Inf ulnar collateral a.

Muscle	Origin	Insertion	Action	Nerve	Artery
Forearm/Wrist					
Flexor Carpi Radialis	Med epicondyle of humerus	Base of 2nd metacarpal bone	↓ wrist Radial ↓	Median n.	Radial a.
Palmaris Longus	Med epicondyle of humerus	Palmar aponeurosis	↓ wrist	Median n.	Volar interosseous a.
Flexor Carpi Ulnaris	Humeral head: med epicondyle of humerus; Ulnar head: med margin olecranon; proximal 2/3 dorsal border of ulna	Pisiform bone	↓ wrist Add wrist	Ulnar n.	Ulnar a.
Flexor Digitorum Superficialis	Humeral head: med epicondyle of humerus; Ulnar head: med side of coronoid process; Radial head: oblique line of radius	Divides into 4 tendons which are inserted into the sides of the 2nd phalanx	↓ PIPs ↓ MCPs ↓ wrist	Median n.	Ulnar a.
Flexor Digitorum Profundus	Proximal 3/4 of volar & med surfaces of body of ulnar	Bases of last phalanges	↓ DIPs ↓ PIPs ↓ MCPs ↓ wrist	Palmar interosseous n. from median n. Branch of ulnar n.	Ulnar a. Volar interosseous a.
Flexor Pollicis Longus	Grooved volar surface of body of the radius	Base of distal phalanx of the thumb	↓ IP digit I ↓ MCP digit I ↓ & add wrist	Palmar interosseous n. from median n.	Radial a.

Muscle	Origin	Insertion	Action	Nerve	Artery
Forearm/Wrist					
Pronator Quadratus	Pronator ridge on distal part of palmar surface of body of ulna; med part of palmar surface of distal 1/4 of ulna	Distal 1/4 of lat border & palmar surface of body of the radius	Pronation	Palmar interosseous n. from median n.	Ulnar & radial a.
Brachioradialis	Proximal 2/3 of lat supracondylar ridge of humerus	Lat side of base of styloid process of radius	✓ elbow	Branch of radial n.	Radial a.
Extensor Carpi Radialis Longus	Distal 1/3 lat supracondylar ridge humerus	Dorsal surface of base of 2nd metacarpal bone—radial side	/ extension Abd wrist	Radial n.	Radial a.
Extensor Carpi Radialis Brevis	Lat epicondyle of humerus	Dorsal surface of base of 3rd metacarpal bone—radial side	/ wrist Abd wrist	Radial n.	Radial a.
Extensor Carpi Ulnaris	Lat epicondyle of humerus	Prominent tubercle on ulnar side of base of metacarpal V	/ wrist Add wrist	Deep radial n.	Ulnar a.
Extensor Digitorum	Lat epicondyle of humerus	2nd & 3rd phalanges of fingers; dorsal surface of distal phalanx	/ PIPs & DIPs; / MCPs / wrist	Deep radial n.	Ulnar a.
Extensor Digiti Minimi	Common extensor tendon	Expansion of ext digitorum tendon on dorsum of 1st phalanx of little finger	/ PIPs, DIPs & MCP digit V	Deep radial n.	Ulnar a.

Muscle	Origin	Insertion	Action	Nerve	Artery
Forearm/Wrist					
Anconeus	Separate tendon from dorsal part of lat epicondyle of humerus	Side of olecranon; proximal 1/4 of dorsal surface of body of ulna	/ elbow	Radial n.	Ulnar a.
Abductor Pollicis Longus	Lat part of dorsal surface of body of ulna	Radial side of base of 1st metacarpal bone	Abd IP, MCP of digit I Abd wrist	Deep radial n.	Radial a.
Extensor Pollicis Brevis	Dorsal surface of body of radius distal to that muscle & interosseous membrane	Base of 1st phalanx of thumb	/ IP, MCP of digit I / wrist	Deep radial n.	Radial a.
Extensor Pollicis Longus	Lat part of mid 1/3 of dorsal surface of body of ulna distal to origin of abductor pollicis longus	Base of last phalanx of thumb	/ IP, MCP of digit I / wrist	Deep radial n.	Radial a.
Extensor Indicis	Dorsal surface of body of ulna below origin of extensor pollicis longus	Joins ulnar side of - tendon of extensor digitorum	/ & add of IP, MCP digit II	Deep radial n.	Radial a.
Supinator	Lat epicondyle of humerus from ridge of ulna	Lat edge of radial tuberosity & oblique line of radius & med surface of radius posteriorly	Supination	Deep radial n.	Radial a.

Muscle	Origin	Insertion	Action	Nerve	Artery
Hand					
Abductor Pollicis Brevis	Transverse carpal ligament, tuberosity of scaphoid, ridge of trapezium	Radial side of base of 1st phalanx thumb	Abd thumb	Median n.	Radial a.
Opponens Pollicis	Ridge of trapezium	Length of metacarpal bone of thumb on radial side	Abd thumb ✓ thumb Med ↻	Median n.	Radial a.
Flexor Pollicis Brevis	Distal ridge of trapezium; ulnar side of 1st metacarpal	Radial side of base of proximal phalanx of thumb; ulnar side of base of 1st phalanx	✓ thumb Add thumb	Median & ulnar n.	Radial a.
Adductor Pollicis	Capitale bone, bases of 2nd & 3rd metacarpals	Ulnar side of base of proximal phalanx of thumb	Add thumb	Deep palmar branch of ulnar n.	Ulnar n.
Palmaris Brevis	Tendinous fasciculi from palmar aponeurosis	Skin on ulnar border of palm of hand	Draws skin mid palm	Ulnar n.	Superficial ulnar a.
Abductor Digiti Minimi	Pisiform bone	Ulnar side of base of 1st phalanx of digit V	Abd digit V ✓ proximal phalanx	Ulnar n.	Ulnar a.
Flexor Digiti Minimi Brevis	Convex surface of hamulus of hamate bone	Ulnar side of base of 1st phalanx of digit V	✓ digit V	Ulnar n.	Ulnar a.

Muscle	Origin	Insertion	Action	Nerve	Artery
Hand					
Opponens Digiti Minimi	Convexity of hamulus of hamate bone	Length of metacarpal bone of digit V along ulnar margin	Abd digit V ✓ digit V Med⤵V	Ulnar n.	Ulnar a.
Lumbricals	Originate from the profundus tendons. 1 & 2: radials sides & palmar surfaces of tendons of digits II & III; 3: contiguous sides of mid & ring fingers; 4: contiguous sides of tendons of ring & little finger	Tendinous expansion of extensor digitorum	✓ MCPs / PIPs & DIPs	1 & 2: median n. 3 & 4: ulnar n.	Median a. Ulnar a.
Interosseous Dorsales	Two heads from adjacent sides of metacarpal bone; all from	Bases of 1st phalanx	Abd—midline (digit III)	Deep palmar (digit III)	Ulnar a. branch n.
Interossei	entire length of metacarpal bones	Side of base of 1st phalanx	Add—midline (digit III) ✓ MCPs / PIPs & DIPs	Deep palmar branch n.	Ulnar a.
Hip					
Psoas Major (Iliopsoas)	Ventral surface of bases and caudal borders of transverse process of	Lesser trochanter of femur	✓ hip ✓ spine in lumbar region	2nd & 3rd lumbar n	Lumbar branch of iliolumbar a.

Muscle	Origin	Insertion	Action	Nerve	Artery
Hip					
	lumbar spine; sides and corresponding intervertebral disks of last thoracic and all lumbar vertebrae				
Psoas Minor (Iliopsoas)	Vertebral margins of T12 & L1, & corresponding disks	Pectineal line; iliopectineal eminence	✓ spine in lumbar region	1st & 2nd lumbar n.	Lumbar branch of iliolumbar a.
Iliacus (Iliopsoas)	Upper 2/3 of iliac fossa; iliac crest	Lesser trochanter of femur	✓ at hip	Femoral n. (muscular branches)	Lumbar branch of iliolumbar a.
Tensor Fasciae Latae (TFL)	Ant part of outer lip of iliac crest; ant border of ilium	Lat part of fascia lata at junction of proximal & mid thirds of thigh (proximal end of iliotibial band)	Tenses TFL ✓ at hip Abd at hip Int ⟲ at hip	Sup gluteal n.	Sup gluteal a.
Gluteus Maximus	Post gluteal line; dorsal surface of sacrum & coccyx	Gluteal tuberosity; lat part of TFL at junction of proximal and mid thirds of thigh (proximal end of iliotibial band)	/ at hip Add at hip Ext ⟲ at hip / lower spine	Inf gluteal n.	Inf gluteal a.

Muscle	Origin	Insertion	Action	Nerve	Artery
Hip					
Gluteus Medius	Outer surface of ilium from iliac crest & post gluteal line above to ant gluteal line below	Lat surface of greater trochanter	Abd at hip Int ↻ at hip	Sup gluteal n.	Sup gluteal a.
Piriformis	Pelvic surface of sacrum between ant sacral foramina & margin of greater sciatic foramen	Upper border of greater trochanter of femur	Ext ↻ at hip Abd at hip	1st & 2nd sacral n.	Sup gluteal a.
Obturator Internus	Margins of obturator foramen; pelvic surface of hip bone; post & sup obturator foramen	Med surface of greater trochanter	Ext ↻ at hip Abd at hip	Obturator n. to obturator internus & gemellus sup	Obturator a. Sup gluteal a.
Gemellus Superior	Outer surface of ischial spine	Med surface of greater trochanter	Ext ↻ at hip	Obturator n. to obturator internus & gemellus sup	Obturator a. Sup gluteal a.
Gemellus Inferior	Upper part of ischial tuberosity	Med surface of greater trochanter	Ext ↻ at hip	Obturator n. to quadratus femoris & gemellus inf	Sup gluteal a.
Quadratus Femoris	Lat margin of ischial tuberosity	Quadrate tubercle of femur; linea quadrata	Add at hip Ext ↻ at hip	Obturator n. to quadratus femoris & gemellus inf	Sup gluteal a.
Obturator Externus	Outer margin of obturator foramen	Trochanteric fossa of femur	Add at hip Ext ↻ at hip	Post branch of obturator n.	Obturator a.

Muscle	Origin	Insertion	Action	Nerve	Artery
Hip/Thigh					
Sartorius	Ant-sup iliac spine; upper half of iliac notch	Upper part of med surface of tibia	✓ at hip Ext↻ at hip ✓ at knee Abd hip (weak)	Muscular branches of femoral n.	Femoral a.
Quadriceps Femoris Rectus Femoris	Ant-inf iliac spine	Tibial Tuberosity	/ at knee ✓ at hip	Muscular branches of femoral n.	Femoral a.
Vastus Lateralis	Lat aspect of the shaft of the femur	Tibial Tuberosity	/ at knee	Muscular branches of femoral n.	Femoral a.
Vastus Medialis	Med aspect of the shaft of the femur	Tibial Tuberosity	/ at knee draws patella medially	Muscular branches of femoral n.	Femoral a.
Vastus Intermedius	Ant aspect of the shaft of the femur	Tibial Tuberosity	/ at knee	Muscular branches of femoral n.	Femoral a.
Gracilis	Lower 1/2 of pubic symphysis; upper 1/2 of pubic arch	Proximal part of med surface of tibia	✓ at knee Int↻ at knee Add at hip	Ant branch of obturator n.	Med femoral circumflex a. (ascending)
Pectineus	Pubic pectineal line & an area of bone ant to it	Line leading from the lesser trochanter to the linea aspera	Add at hip ✓ at hip Int↻ hip	Muscular branches of femoral & obturator n.	Med femoral circumflex a.

Hip/Thigh

Muscle	Origin	Insertion	Action	Nerve	Artery
Adductor Longus	Ant portion of pubis in angle between crest & symphysis	Mid part of linea aspera	Add at hip / ✓ at hip	Ant branch of obturator n.	Profunda femoris a.
Adductor Brevis	Ext surface of inf ramus of pubis	Proximal part of linea aspera	Add at hip / ✓ at hip	Ant branch of obturator n.	Mid femoral circumflex a.
Adductor Magnus	Pubic arch & ischial tuberosity	Oblique line along entire shaft of the femur	Add at hip / ✓ hip (upper) / hip (lower)	Post branch of obturator & sciatic n.	Profunda femoris & med femoris circumflex a.
Biceps Femoris	Long head: from ischial tuberosity; Short head: lat lip of linea aspera; lat supra-condylar line of femur	Head of fibula, lat condyle of tibia, deep fascia on lat side of leg	✓ at knee / at hip Ext ⟳ knee (semiflexed)	Sciatic n. tibial branch to long head; peroneal branch to short head	Profunda femoris a.
Semitendinous	Upper & mid impression of ischial tuberosity (with tendon of the biceps femoris)	Proximal part of ant border & med surface of the tibia	✓ at knee / at hip Int ⟲ knee (semiflexed)	Sciatic n.	Perforating branch profunda femoris a.
Semimembranous	Proximal & lat facet of ischial tuberosity	Med-post surface of med condyle of tibia	✓ at knee / at hip Int ⟲ knee (semiflexed)	Sciatic n.	Perforating branch profunda femoris a.

Muscle	Origin	Insertion	Action	Nerve	Artery
Leg					
Tibialis Anterior	Lat surface of shaft of tibia; med aspect of fibula; ant interosseous membrane	Med & plantar surface of med cuniform bone; base of 1st metatarsal bone	Dorsiflexion inversion	Deep peroneal n.	Ant tibial a.
Popliteus	Lat condyle of femur	Triangular area on post surface of tibia above sdeal line	✓ at knee Int ↻ at knee	Tibial n. (med & int popliteal)	Post tibial a.
Leg/Foot					
Extensor Hallucis Longus	Lat surface of shaft of tibia; med aspect of fibula; ant interosseous membrane	Base of distal phalanx of great toe	/ MTP & IP Dorsiflexion	Deep peroneal n. (ant tibial)	Ant tibial a.
Extensor Digitorum Longus (EDL)	Lat surface of shaft of tibia; med aspect of fibula; ant - interosseous membrane	Dorsal surface of mid & distal phalanges of lat 4 digits	/ IPs digits II to V Dorsiflexion	Deep peroneal n. (ant tibial)	Ant tibial a.
Extensor Digitorum Brevis (EDB)	Proximal & lat surface of calcaneus; lat talo-calcaneal ligament	1st tendon dorsal surface of base of proximal phalanx of hallux; other 3 tendons lat sides of tendons of EDL	/ IPs	Deep peroneal n.	Ant tibial a.

Muscle	Origin	Insertion	Action	Nerve	Artery
Leg/Foot					
Flexor Digitorum Longus	Post surface of shaft of tibia; post aspect of fibula; post interosseous membrane	Plantar surface of base of distal phalanx of lat 4 digits	✓ digits II to V Plantar-flexion	Tibial n. (med & int popliteal)	Post tibial a.
Flexor Hallucis Longus	Post surface of shaft of tibia; post aspect of fibula; post interosseous membrane	Base of distal phalanx of hallux	✓ digit I Plantarflexion	Tibial n. (med & int popliteal)	Post tibial a.
Tibialis Posterior	Post surface of shaft of tibia; post aspect of fibula; post interosseous membrane	Tuberosity of navicular; plantar surface of cuniform bones; plantar surface of base of 2nd, 3rd & 4th metatarsals, cuboid, sustentaculum tali	Plantarflexion Inversion	Tibial n. (med & int popliteal)	Post tibial a.
Peroneus Tertius	Lat surface of shaft of tibia; med aspect of fibula; ant interosseous membrane	Dorsal surface of base of 5th metatarsal bone	Dorsiflexion Eversion	Deep peroneal n. (ant tibial)	Ant tibial a.
Peroneus Longus	Lat condyle of tibia; head & upper 2/3 of lat surface of fibula	Lat side of med cuniform bone, base of 1st metatarsal bone	Plantarflexion Eversion	Superficial peroneal n. (musculocutaneous)	Peroneal a.

Muscle	Origin	Insertion	Action	Nerve	Artery
Leg/Foot					
Peroneus Brevis	Lower 2/3 of lat surface of fibula	Lat side of base of 5th metatarsal bone	Plantarflexion Eversion	Superficial peroneal n. (musculocutaneous)	Peroneal a.
Gastrocnemius	Med head: med condyle & adjacent part of femur; capsule of knee; Long head: lat condyle & adjacent part of femur; capsule of knee	Calcaneus by the calcaneal tendon	Plantarflexion ✓ at knee	Tibial n. (med popliteal)	Popliteal a.
Soleus	Post surface of head & proximal 1/3 of shaft of fibula; mid 1/3 of med border of tibia	Calcaneus by the calcaneal tendon	Plantarflexion	Tibial n. (med popliteal)	Post tibial a.
Plantaris	Lat supracondylar line of femur	Med side of post part of calcaneus	Plantarflexion	Tibial n. (med popliteal)	Post tibial a.
Foot					
Quadratus Plantae	Med head: med surface of calcaneus & med border of long plantar ligament; Lat head: lat border of plantar surface of calcaneus & lat border of long plantar ligament	Attached to tendons of flexor digitorum longus	✓ last IP digits II to V	Lat plantar n.	Lat plantar a.

Muscle	Origin	Insertion	Action	Nerve	Artery
Foot					
Lumbricals (4)	Tendons of flexor digitorum longus	Tendons of EDL & interossei into bases of last phalanges of digits II-V	✓ MP joints / IP joints	Med plantar n. Deep lat plantar n.	Med plantar a.

Key:
✓ flexion
/ extension
↻ rotation
▼ depression, downward, caudal
▲ elevation, upward, cephalic
◆ outward, expand
n. = nerve
a. = artery
Lat = lateral
Med = medial
Ext = external
Int = internal
Sup = superior
Inf = inferior

Ant = anterior
Post = posterior
Min = minimal
MTP = metatarsophalangeal
MCP = metacarpophalangeal
IP = interphalangeal
PIP = proximal interphalangeal
DIP = distal interphalangeal
Opp = opposite
Abd = abduction
Add = adduction
Mid = middle

Reprinted with permission from Bottomley J. *Quick Reference Dictionary for Physical Therapy.* Thorofare, NJ: SLACK Incorporated; 2000.

Manual Muscle Testing

This section provides an overview of muscle testing procedures for the major muscle groups of the extremities. Origin, insertion, action, and nerve innervation are provided in the previous appendix. *When picture angle allows, an arrow depicts direction of patient's movement.*

Hip, Thigh, Knee

Iliopsoas

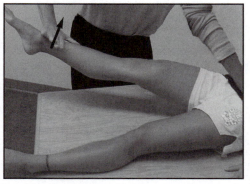

Patient positioning: Supine with hip externally rotated, slightly abducted and flexed.
Patient action: Hip flexion.
Examiner positioning: Applies pressure to the distal leg in an extension and abduction direction.
Examiner stabilization: Stabilizes opposite hip over the ASIS.

Internal Rotators: Tensor Fascia Latae, Gluteus Medius

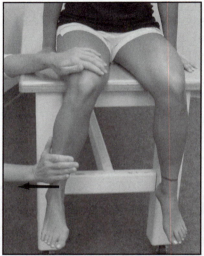

Patient positioning: Seated with hip and knee flexed to 90 degrees.

Patient action: Internally rotates hip against examiner stabilization. This is accomplished by moving the lower leg laterally thereby internally rotating the thigh at the hip.

Examiner positioning: Applies pressure to the lateral aspect of the distal lower leg in a medial (adduction) direction while the patient resists motion.

Examiner stabilization: Stabilizes the leg medially at the knee.

External Rotators: Obturators, Piriformis, Gemelli,
Quadratus Femoris

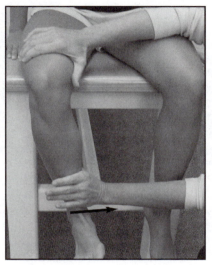

Patient positioning: Seated with hip and knee flexed to 90 degrees.

Patient action: Externally rotates hip against examiner stabilization. This is accomplished by moving the lower leg medially thereby externally rotating the thigh at the hip.

Examiner positioning: Applies pressure to the medial aspect of the distal lower leg in a lateral (abduction) direction while the patient resists motion.

Examiner stabilization: Stabilizes the leg laterally at the knee.

Adductor Longus, Adductor Magnus, Adductor Brevis

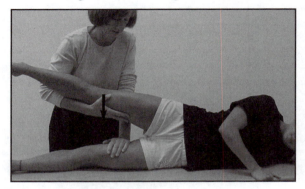

Patient positioning: Side-lying.
Patient action: Hip adduction.
Examiner positioning: Passively abduct upper leg. Stabilize lower bottom leg to table and resist patient's attempt to adduct upper leg back toward table.
Examiner stabilization: Stabilize legs just proximal to the knee.

Lateral Hamstrings: Biceps Femoris

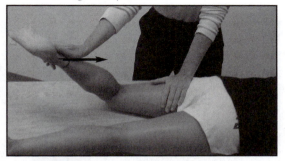

Patient positioning: Prone with knee flexed approx 50 degrees, hip externally rotated and tibia externally rotated.
Patient action: Knee flexion.
Examiner positioning: Grasp distal lower leg maintaining external tibial rotation and resist patient's knee flexion.
Examiner stabilization: Usually not necessary. If patient's hip flexes and pelvis comes off the table, stabilize pelvis by applying pressure over the PSIS.

Medial Hamstrings: Semimembranosus, Semitendinosus

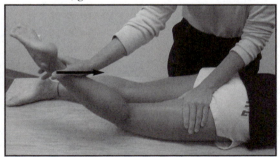

Patient positioning: Prone with knee flexed approx 50 degrees, hip internally rotated and tibia internally rotated.
Patient action: Knee flexion.
Examiner positioning: Grasp distal lower leg maintaining interal tibial rotation and resist patient's knee flexion.
Examiner stabilization: Usually not necessary. If patient's hip flexes and pelvis comes off the table, stabilize pelvis by applying pressure over the PSIS.

Gluteus Maximus

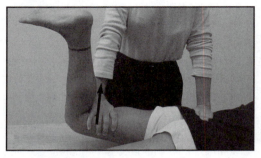

Patient positioning: Prone with knee flexed to at least 90 degrees.
Patient action: Hip extension with knee flexed.
Examiner positioning: Applies pressure to the distal thigh in a downward (flexion) direction.
Examiner stabilization: Stabilize the pelvis to the table at the PSIS.

Gluteus Medius

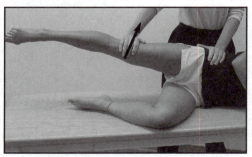

Patient positioning: Side-lying with hip abducted and internally rotated. Bottom leg is positioned with knee and hip flexed.
Patient action: Resist examiner's attempt to adduct thigh.
Examiner positioning: Applies pressure at lateral knee in a downward (adduction) direction.
Examiner stabilization: Stabilize trunk at the iliac crest.

Gluteus Minimus

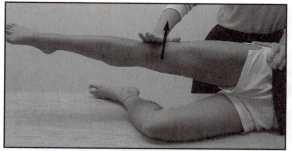

Patient positioning: Side-lying with hip abducted and externally rotated, knee extended. Bottom leg is positioned with knee and hip flexed.

Patient action: Resist examiner's attempt to adduct thigh.

Examiner positioning: Applies pressure at lateral knee in a downward (adduction) direction.

Examiner stabilization: Stabilize trunk at the iliac crest.

Tensor Fasciae Lata

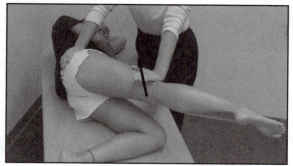

Patient positioning: A position in-between supine and side-lying with hip flexed and abducted and internally rotated, knee extended. Bottom leg is positioned with knee and hip flexed.

Patient action: Abduction and flexion of hip.

Examiner positioning: Applies pressure at lateral knee diagonally in adduction and extension directions.

Examiner stabilization: Stabilize trunk at the iliac crest.

Sartorius

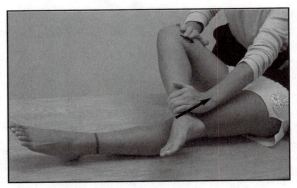

Patient positioning: Supine with hip flexed, abducted and externally rotated, knee flexed approximately 80 degrees.

Patient action: Combined motions of flexion, abduction, external rotation while flexing knee.

Examiner positioning: Applies resistance to the patient's combined movements of hip flexion, abduction, and external rotation while simultaneously resisting knee flexion.

Examiner stabilization: Stabilize upper leg anteriorly on the distal thigh just above the knee and at the distal end of the lower leg by grasping the ankle.

Rectus Femoris (as hip flexor)

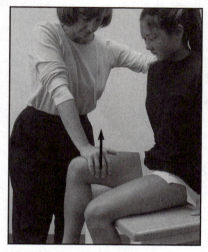

Patient positioning: Seated with knee flexed to 90 degrees.
Patient action: Hip flexion while maintaining knee flexion.
Examiner positioning: Applies pressure to the distal thigh just above the knee resisting hip flexion.
Examiner stabilization: Stabilize the trunk at the shoulder.

Rectus Femoris (as knee extensor)

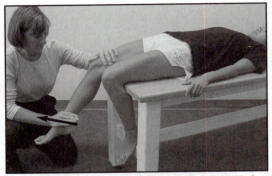

Patient positioning: Supine with knees flexed to 90 degrees (legs hanging over edge of table).
Patient action: Knee extension.
Examiner positioning: Applies pressure to the distal lower leg resisting patient's knee joint extension.
Examiner stabilization: n/a

Vastus Lateralis, Vastus Medialis, Vastus Intermedius

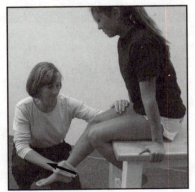

Patient positioning: Seated with hips and knees flexed to 90 degrees (legs hanging over table).
Patient action: Knee extension.
Examiner positioning: Applies pressure over distal lower leg resisting patient's knee joint extension.
Examiner stabilization: n/a

Lower Leg, Ankle, Foot

Gastrocnemius

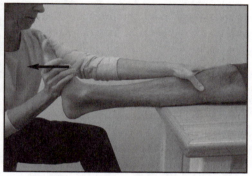

Patient positioning: Supine or seated with knee extended.
Patient action: Plantar flexion.
Examiner positioning: Applies pressure to the plantar surface of the foot near metatarsal heads resisting patient's plantar flexion.
Examiner stabilization: Stabilizes foot by grasping the calcaneus; patient may grasp table for support.

Soleus

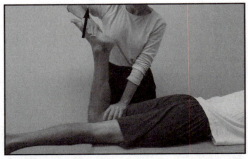

Patient positioning: Prone with knee flexed to 90 degrees.
Patient action: Plantar flexion.
Examiner positioning: Applies pressure to the plantar surface of the foot near metatarsal heads resisting patient's plantar flexion.
Examiner stabilization: Stabilizes lower leg.

Tibialis Posterior

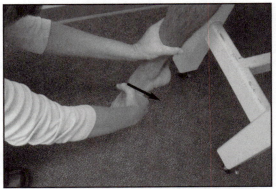

Patient positioning: Seated with leg hanging over edge of table with foot everted.
Patient action: Plantar flexion/inversion.
Examiner positioning: Grasps medial aspect of foot and resists patient's plantar flexion/inversion.
Examiner stabilization: Stabilizes lower leg.

Peroneus Longus, Peroneus Brevis

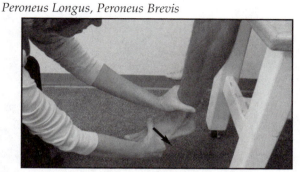

Patient positioning: Seated with leg hanging over edge of table with foot inverted.
Patient action: Plantar flexion/eversion.
Examiner positioning: Grasps lateral aspect of foot and resists patient's plantar flexion/eversion.
Examiner stabilization: Stabilizes lower leg.

Peroneus Tertius

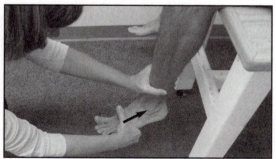

Patient positioning: Seated with leg hanging over edge of table with foot inverted.
Patient action: Dorsiflexion/eversion.
Examiner positioning: Grasps lateral aspect of foot and resists patient's dorsiflexion/eversion.
Examiner stabilization: Stabilizes lower leg.

Tibialis Anterior

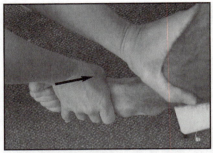

Patient positioning: Seated with leg hanging over edge of table with foot inverted.
Patient action: Dorsiflexion/inversion.
Examiner positioning: Grasps medial aspect of foot and resists patient's dorsiflexion/inversion.
Examiner stabilization: Stabilizes lower leg.

Extensor Digitorum Longus

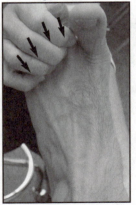

Patient positioning: Seated or supine with foot slightly plantar flexed.
Patient action: Extension of the four lateral toes.
Examiner positioning: Applies pressure to the dorsal aspect of the four lateral toes in a flexion direction.
Examiner stabilization: Stabilize foot at the calcaneus in slight plantar flexion.

Extensor Hallucis Longus

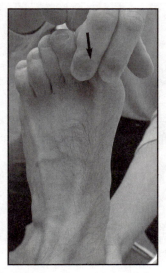

Patient positioning: Seated or supine with foot in neutral and great toe extended.
Patient action: Resists examiner's attempt to flex great toe.
Examiner positioning: Applies pressure to the dorsal aspect of great toe to attempting to move toe into flexion.
Examiner stabilization: Stabilize foot at the calcaneus in neutral position.

Flexor Digitorum Longus

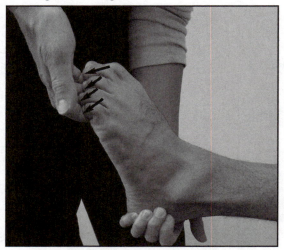

Patient positioning: Supine.
Patient action: Flexion of four lateral toes.
Examiner positioning: Applies pressure to plantar surface of four lateral toes.
Examiner stabilization: Stabilize forefoot.

Flexor Hallucis Longus

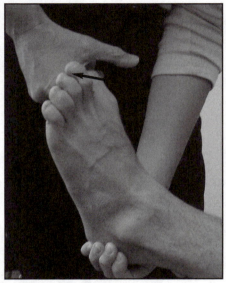

Patient positioning: Supine.
Patient action: Flexion of great toe.
Examiner positioning: Applies pressure to plantar surface of great toe.
Examiner stabilization: Stabilize forefoot.

Shoulder, Shoulder Girdle

Coracobrachialis

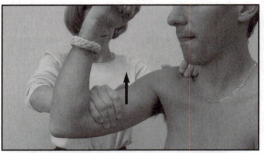

Patient positioning: Seated or supine with elbow fully flexed and shoulder flexed to approx 80 degrees.
Patient action: Shoulder flexion.
Examiner positioning: Applies pressure at mid-bicep resisting shoulder flexion.
Examiner stabilization: Stabilize trunk from moving if patient is seated.

Deltoid (anterior)

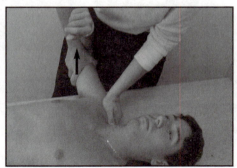

Patient positioning: Supine with shoulder internally rotated and abducted to 90 degrees, elbow flexed to 90 degrees.
Patient action: Horizontal adduction.
Examiner positioning: Applies pressure to the distal humerus resisting patient's horizontal adduction.
Examiner stabilization: Stabilizes the trunk to the table by applying pressure over the shoulder joint.

Deltoid (middle)

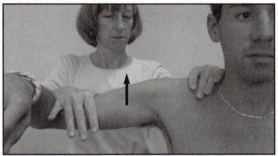

Patient positioning: Seated with shoulder internally rotated and abducted to approximately 70 degrees, elbow flexed to 90 degrees.
Patient action: Abduction of the shoulder joint.
Examiner positioning: Applies pressure to the distal humerus resisting patient's abduction.
Examiner stabilization: Stabilizes the patient at the shoulder.

Deltoid (posterior)

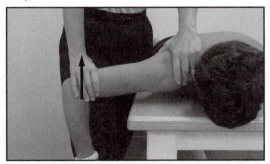

Patient positioning: Prone with shoulder internally rotated and abducted to 90 degrees, elbow flexed to 90 degrees.
Patient action: Horizontal abduction.
Examiner positioning: Applies pressure to the distal humerus resisting patient's horizontal abduction.
Examiner stabilization: Stabilizes the trunk to the table by applying pressure over the shoulder joint.

Pectoralis Major

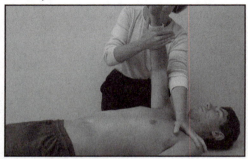

Patient positioning: Supine with shoulder internally rotated and flexed to 90 degrees, elbow extended.

Patient action: Horizontal flexion for upper fibers, diagonally toward opposite hip for lower fibers.

Examiner positioning: Grasp arm distal to the elbow and resist patient's horizontal or diagonal movement.

Examiner stabilization: Stabilize trunk to table by applying pressure to the opposite shoulder when testing the upper fibers and pressure to the opposite hip when testing the lower fibers.

Pectoralis Minor

Patient positioning: Supine with arms at side.

Patient action: Protraction.

Examiner positioning: Apply pressure to the anterior aspect of the shoulders resisting patient's protraction.

Examiner stabilization: Stabilize shoulder to the table.

Serratus Anterior

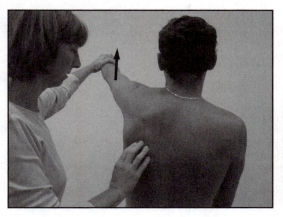

Patient positioning: Sitting with shoulder slightly internally rotated, flexed approximately 125 degrees, and abducted approximately 45 degrees.

Patient action: Resist examiner's attempt to extend arm.

Examiner positioning: Applies downward (extension) force to the upper arm proximal to the elbow. Palpate for patient's inability to stabilized the scapula.

Examiner stabilization: One hand is placed on the lateral border of the scapula to track the movement of the scapula.

Subscapularis, Pectoralis Major, Teres Major, Latissimus Dorsi (internal rotators)

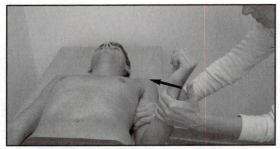

Patient positioning: Supine with humerus at the patient's side, elbow flexed to 90 degrees.
Patient action: Internal rotation of the shoulder joint.
Examiner positioning: Applies pressure distally to the ventral side of the patient's arm near the wrist resisting internal shoulder rotation.
Examiner stabilization: Stabilize the elbow to the side of the patient's body.

Teres Major

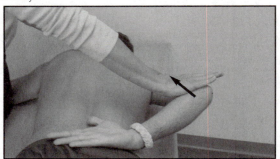

Patient positioning: Prone with back of hand on posterior iliac crest creating an internally rotated position.
Patient action: Extension and adduction of humerus while internally rotated.
Examiner positioning: Applies pressure to the elbow resisting patient's extension and adduction.
Examiner stabilization: Stabilize trunk to table by applying pressure to the shoulder girdle.

Teres Minor, Infraspinatus (external rotators)

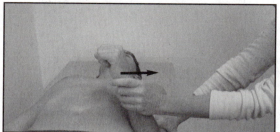

Patient positioning: Supine with humerus at the patient's side, elbow flexed to 90 degrees.
Patient action: External rotation of the shoulder joint.
Examiner positioning: Applies pressure distally to the dorsal side of the patient's arm near the wrist resisting external shoulder rotation.
Examiner stabilization: Stabilize the elbow medially at the side of the patient's body.

Latissimus Dorsi

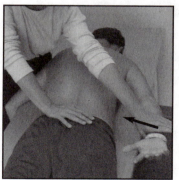

Patient positioning: Prone with shoulder extended slightly past neutral, abducted approximately 30 degrees, and internally rotated.
Patient action: Shoulder joint adduction.
Examiner positioning: Grasps forearm distally and resists patient's adduction.
Examiner stabilization: Stabilize trunk by applying pressure to the sacrum.

Levator Scapulae

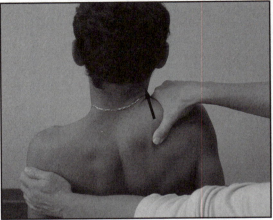

Patient positioning: Seated with shoulders retracted.
Patient action: Shoulder girdle elevation while retracted.
Examiner positioning: Applies pressure to the superior aspect of the shoulder joint over the acromion process and resists patient's elevation of shoulder girdle.
Examiner stabilization: Stabilize the opposite side at the shoulder to keep patient from laterally flexing at the trunk.

Upper Trapezius

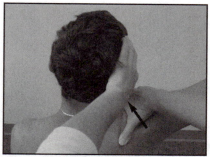

Patient positioning: Seated with shoulder internally rotated, abducted to 90 degrees upward rotated shoulder girdle, and head extended and laterally flexed toward shoulder.

Patient action: Shoulder girdle upward rotation.

Examiner positioning: Applies pressure to the head and superior aspect of the shoulder and attempts to "pry" apart.

Examiner stabilization: Stabilize the head.

Lower Trapezius

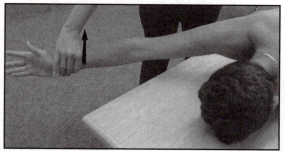

Patient positioning: Prone with shoulder externally rotated and abducted approximately 130 degrees.

Patient action: Flexion, abduction of the shoulder: resist examiner's attempt to move arm in a downward direction.

Examiner positioning: Apply pressure to the distal forearm just above the wrist in a downward direction. Observe patient's scapula.

Examiner stabilization: Not necessary.

Rhomboids, Middle Trapezius

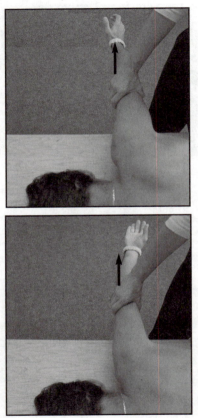

Patient positioning: Prone with shoulder abducted to 90 degrees. The shoulder is positioned in external rotation for middle trapezius and internal rotation for rhomboids.
Patient action: Resists examiner's attempt to horizontal adduct.
Examiner positioning: Applies pressure at the distal forearm in a downward direction (ie, toward floor).
Examiner stabilization: Stabilize trunk to table at opposite shoulder.

Elbow, Forearm, Wrist

Extensor Carpi Radialis Longus and Brevis

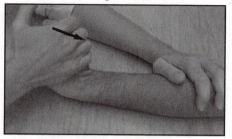

Patient positioning: Forearm pronated, elbow nearly extended, loosely closed fist. Performed with elbow flexed for brevis.
Patient action: Extends and radially deviates.
Examiner positioning: Grasps wrist and applies pressure to resist extension and radial deviation.
Examiner stabilization: Stabilizes forearm distally.

Extensor Carpi Ulnaris

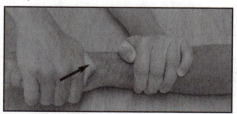

Patient positioning: Forearm pronated, elbow nearly extended, loosely closed fist.
Patient action: Extends and ulnar deviates.
Examiner positioning: Grasps wrist and applies pressure to resist extension and ulnar deviation.
Examiner stabilization: Stabilizes forearm distally.

Flexor Carpi Radialis

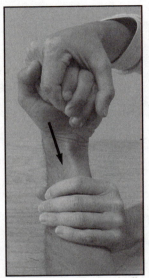

Patient positioning: Forearm supinated, elbow 90 degrees or greater, wrist in slight ulnar deviation.
Patient action: Flexes and radial deviates.
Examiner positioning: Grasps hand and applies pressure to resist flexion and radial deviation.
Examiner stabilization: Stabilizes forearm distally.

Flexor Carpi Ulnaris

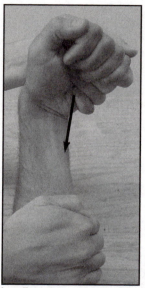

Patient positioning: Forearm supinated, elbow 90 degrees or greater, wrist in slight radial deviation.
Patient action: Flexes and ulnar deviates.
Examiner positioning: Grasps hand and applies pressure to resist flexion and ulnar deviation.
Examiner stabilization: Stabilizes forearm distally.

Pronator Quadratus

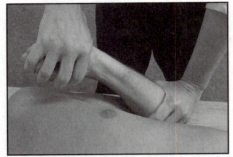

Patient positioning: Supine with elbow maximally flexed, forearm in neutral position.
Patient action: Pronation of the forearm.
Examiner positioning: Grasps patient's wrist and resists patient's pronation.
Examiner stabilization: Stabilizes elbow up against the patient's body.

Pronator Teres

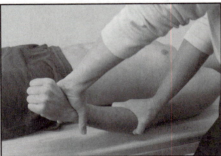

Patient positioning: Supine with elbow approximately 165 degrees, forearm in neutral position.
Patient action: Pronation of the forearm.
Examiner positioning: Grasps patient's wrist and resists patient's pronation.
Examiner stabilization: Stabilizes elbow up against the patient's body.

Supinator

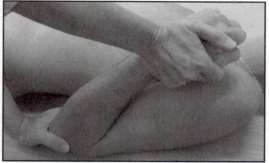

Patient positioning: Supine with elbow maximally flexed, forearm in neutral position.
Patient action: Supination of the forearm.
Examiner positioning: Grasps patient's wrist and resists patient's supination.
Examiner stabilization: Stabilizes elbow.

Biceps Brachii

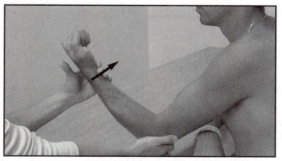

Patient positioning: Elbow flexed to approximately 100 degrees, forearm supinated, elbow resting in examiner's hand.
Patient action: Elbow flexion while supinated.
Examiner positioning: Applies pressure to the distal forearm resisting patient elbow flexion.
Examiner stabilization: Stabilizes upper arm at the elbow.

Brachialis

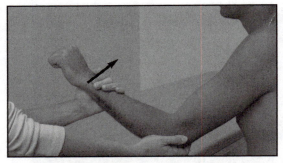

Patient positioning: Elbow flexed to approximately 100 degrees, forearm pronated, elbow resting in examiner's hand.
Patient action: Elbow flexion while pronated.
Examiner positioning: Applies pressure to the distal forearm resisting patient elbow flexion.
Examiner stabilization: Stabilizes upper arm at the elbow.

Brachioradialis

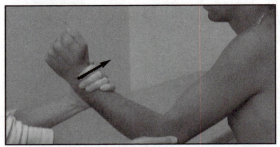

Patient positioning: Elbow flexed to approximately 100 degrees, forearm in neutral position, elbow resting in examiner's hand.
Patient action: Elbow flexion, neutral forearm position.
Examiner positioning: Applies pressure to the distal forearm resisting patient elbow flexion.
Examiner stabilization: Stabilizes upper arm at the elbow.

Triceps

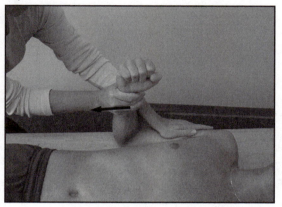

Patient positioning: Supine with elbow flexed to 90 degrees, forearm in neutral position.
Patient action: Extends elbow.
Examiner positioning: Grasps forearm distally at the wrist and resists patient elbow extension.
Examiner stabilization: Stabilizes upper arm against patient's body and against table.

Hand

Abductor Pollicus Longus

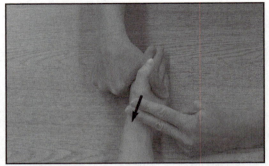

Patient positioning: Forearm in neutral position, thumb flexed at the metacarpophalangeal joint, resting in examiner's hand.
Patient action: Abduction of the carpometacarpal joint.
Examiner positioning: Applies pressure to the metacarpal and resists patient's abduction.
Examiner stabilization: Stabilizes the hand.

Abductor Pollicus Brevis

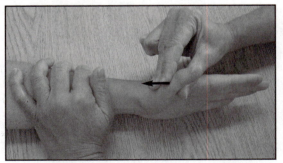

Patient positioning: Forearm and hand in neutral position, forearm slightly supinated.
Patient action: Thumb abduction; movement toward forearm.
Examiner positioning: Applies pressure at the proximal phalanx; resists patient from moving into abduction.
Examiner stabilization: Stabilizes patient's hand.

Adductor Pollicis

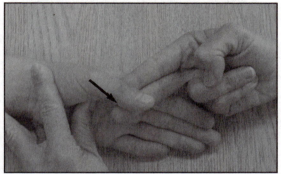

Patient positioning: Hand resting on table, forearm supinated.

Patient action: Adduction of thumb (movement toward 1st metacarpal).

Examiner positioning: Applies pressure at the proximal phalanx; resists patient adduction.

Examiner stabilization: Stabilizes the hand against the table at the metacarpophalangeal joints.

Extensor Pollicis Brevis

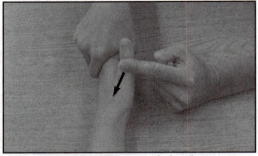

Patient positioning: Forearm neutral, hand resting on table, thumb slightly flexed at the metacarpophalangeal joint.
Patient action: Extension of the metacarpophalangeal joint and abduction of the carpometacarpal joint.
Examiner positioning: Extension of the metacarpophalangeal joint and abduction of the carpometacarpal joint.
Examiner stabilization: Stabilizes patient hand.

Extensor Pollicis Longus

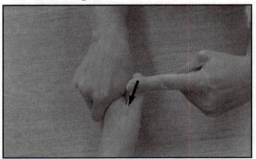

Patient positioning: Forearm slightly pronated, hand resting on table.
Patient action: Extension of the caropmetacarpal, metacarpophalnageal, and interphalangeal joints of the thumb.
Examiner positioning: Applies pressure to the distal phalanx of the thumb and resists patient's extension.
Examiner stabilization: Stabilizes patient hand.

Flexor Pollicis Brevis

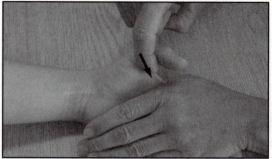

Patient positioning: Forearm supinated, resting in examiner's hand.

Patient action: Flexion of the metacarpophalangeal joint of the thumb.

Examiner positioning: Applies pressure to the proximal phalanx resisting patient flexion.

Examiner stabilization: Stabilizes hand at the wrist.

Flexor Pollicis Longus

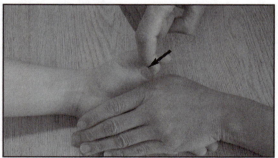

Patient positioning: Forearm supinated, hand resting on table.

Patient action: Flexion of the interphalangeal joint of the thumb.

Examiner positioning: Applies pressure to the distal phalanx and resists patient's flexion of the interphalangeal joint.

Examiner stabilization: Stabilizes the proximal phalanx of the thumb.

Extensor Digitorum Test I

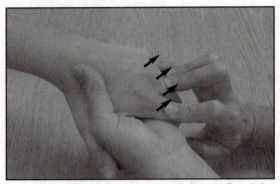

Patient positioning: Forearm pronated, fingers flexed, hand resting on table.

Patient action: Extension of the metacarpophalangeal joints of the fingers.

Examiner positioning: Applies pressure to the proximal phalanges at the proximal interphalangeal joints resisting patient's extension.

Examiner stabilization: Stabilizes the forearm at the wrist.

Extensor Digitorum Test II

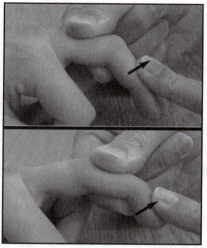

Patient positioning: Forearm pronated, hand resting in examiner's hand.

Patient action: Extension of the proximal interphalangeal (PIP) and distal interphalangeal (DIP) joints of each finger.

Examiner positioning: Applies pressure to the distal phalanx of each finger resisting extension of the PIP and DIP joint of each finger.

Examiner stabilization: Stabilizes the middle phalanx of each finger.

Extensor Indicis*

Extensor Digiti Minimi (hand)*

*Impossible to discriminate from extensor digitorum—see previous examples

Flexor Digitorum Profundus

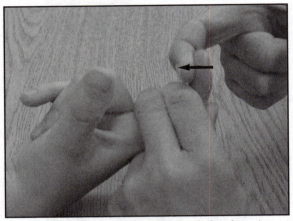

Patient positioning: Forearm supinated, hand resting on table.

Patient action: Flexion of the DIP joints of the four fingers.

Examiner positioning: Applies pressure to the distal phalanx of each finger resisting DIP flexion.

Examiner stabilization: Stabilizes the middle phalanx of each finger.

Flexor Digitorum Superficialis

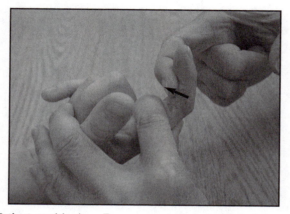

Patient positioning: Forearm supinated, hand resting on table.

Patient action: Flexion of the PIP joints of the four fingers.

Examiner positioning: Applies pressure to the middle phalanx and resists PIP flexion.

Examiner stabilization: Stabilizes the proximal phalanx of each finger.

APPENDIX 7

Normal Joint Ranges of Motion

Cervical Spine

Flexion	0 to (45-90 degrees)
Extension	0 to (50-70 degrees)
Lateral flexion	0 to (20-45 degrees)
Rotation	0 to (60-90 degrees)

Lumbar Spine

Flexion	0 to (40-60 degrees)
Extension	0 to (20-35 degrees)
Lateral flexion	0 to (15-20 degrees)
Rotation	0 to (3-12 degrees)

Shoulder

Flexion	0 to (167-180 degrees)
Extension	0 to (45-62 degrees)
Abduction	0 to (170-184 degrees)
Internal rotation	0 to (69-90 degrees)
External rotation	0 to (90-104 degrees)
Horizontal flexion (adduction)	0 to (30-45 degrees)
Horizontal extension (abduction)	0 to (135-140 degrees)

Elbow

Flexion	0 to (135-150 degrees)
Pronation	0 to (75-90 degrees)
Supination	0 to (70-90 degrees)

Wrist

Flexion	0 to (60-90 degrees)
Extension	0 to (50-90 degrees)
Abduction	0 to (40-45 degrees)
Adduction	0 to (15-30 degrees)

Hand

Fingers 2-5
    MCP
        Flexion   0 to (85-90 degrees)
        Extension   0 to (30-45 degrees)
    PIP
        Flexion   0 to (100-115 degrees)
        Extension   0 degrees
    DIP
        Flexion   0 to (80-90 degrees)
        Extension   0 to 20 degrees
        Abduction   0 to (20-30 degrees)
Thumb
    CM
        Flexion   0 to 50 degrees
        Extension   0 degrees
    MCP
        Flexion   0 to 55 degrees
        Extension   0 degrees
    IP
        Flexion   0 to 90 degrees
        Extension   0 to 5 degrees
        Abduction   0 to 70 degrees
        Adduction   0 to 30 degrees

Hip

Flexion	0 to (100-130 degrees)
Extension	0 to (15-50 degrees)
Abduction	0 to (40-50 degrees)

Adduction	0 to (15-45 degrees)
Internal rotation	0 to (30-45 degrees)
External rotation	0 to (35-50 degrees)
Horizontal flexion (adduction)	0 to 40 degrees
Horizontal extension (abduction)	0 to (50-90 degrees)

Knee

Flexion	0 to (120-145 degrees)

Ankle

Plantar flexion	0 to (40-65 degrees)
Dorsiflexion	0 to (10-30 degrees)
Inversion	0 to (30-50 degrees)
Eversion	0 to (15-25 degrees)
Supination	0 to (45-60 degrees)
Pronation	0 to (20-30 degrees)

Foot

MTP flexion (great toe)	0 to 45 degrees
MTP flexion (toes 2-5)	0 to 40 degrees
MTP extension (great toe)	0 to 70 degrees
MTP extension (toes 2-5)	0 to 40 degrees
IP flexion (great toe)	0 to 90 degrees
IP extension (great toe)	0 degrees
DIP flexion (toes 2-5)	0 to 60 degrees
PIP flexion (toes 2-5)	0 to 35 degrees
DIP extension (toes 2-5)	0 to 30 degrees
PIP extension (toes 2-5)	0 degrees

APPENDIX 8

Cranial Nerves and Assessment

Number	Nerve	Function	Assessment
I	Olfactory	Smell	Assess recognition of common smells (grass, sports drink, liniment/balm, etc).
II	Optic	Visual acuity, reaction to light	Assess visual field: assess one eye at a time. Patient focuses on examiner and states when examiner's finger is in visual field. Examiner starts near the edge of visual field and moves finger slowly toward center of patient's vision. Eyes react to light. Patient can focus near and distant vision.
III	Oculomotor	Eye movement	Assess patient's ability to move eyes upward, downward, and medially.
IV	Trochlear	Inferiolateral eye movement	Assess patient's ability to move eyes downward and laterally.

Number	Nerve	Function	Assessment
V	Trigeminal	Facial sensation	Assess sense of touch on the face; patient clenches teeth.
VI	Abducens	Lateral eye movement	Assess patient's ability to move eyes laterally.
VII	Facial	Facial movements, taste	Ask patient to perform a number of facial movements (eg, eyes closed, purse lips, smile, raise eyebrows, frown, blow-out cheeks, etc; identify common tastes).
VIII	Vestibulocochlear	Hearing/balance	Can hear fingers rubbing together near ear, tapping, etc; balance and coordination tests.

Number	Nerve	Function	Assessment
IX	Glossopharyngeal	Taste, tongue movements	Can swallow; may check gag reflex.
X	Vagus	Breathing, tasting, swallowing	Same as above.
XI	Accessory	Sternocleidomastoid and trapezius motor function	Assess neck flexion, shrug shoulders.
XII	Hypoglosseal	Muscles of the tongue	Assess tongue movements.

APPENDIX 9

Concussion Grading

Grade	Cantu	Colorado	American Academy of Neurology
1	no LOC amnesia < 30 min	no LOC amnesia < 30 min	concussion symptoms < 15 min, no amnesia
2	LOC < 5 min amnesia > 30 min	LOC < 5 min amnesia > 30 min	concussion symptoms > 15 min
3	LOC > 5 min amnesia > 24 hr	any loss of consciousness	any loss of consciousness

Comparison of Return to Play Guidelines

Grade	Cantu	Colorado	American Academy of Neurology
Grade 1			
1st concussion	When asymptomatic for 1 week	Asymptomatic for 20 min	Asymptomatic for 15 min
2nd concussion	2 weeks when asymptomatic for 1 week	When asymptomatic for 1 week	When asymptomatic for 1 week
3rd concussion	Terminate season; may return next season if asymptomatic	May return in 3 months	—
Grade 2			
1st concussion	When asymptomatic for 1 week	When asymptomatic for 1 week	When asymptomatic for 1 week
2nd concussion	Min. 1 month, may return; if symptomatic for 1 week, consider termination	When asymptomatic for 1 month	When asymptomatic for 2 weeks

Grade	Cantu	Colorado	American Academy of Neurology
3rd concussion	Terminate season; may return next season if asymptomatic	Terminate season; may return next season	—
Grade 3			
1st concussion	Min. 1 month, may return if asymptomatic for 1 week	Immediate referral, return 1 month if asymptomatic for 2 weeks	Immediate referral, return when asymptomatic for 1 week
2nd concussion	Terminate season; may return next season if asymptomatic	Terminate season	When asymptomatic for 1 month

Cantu RC. Posttraumatic retrograde and anterograde amnesia: pathophysiology and implications in grading and safe return to play. *Journal of Athletic Training.* 2001;36:3.

Harmon KG. Assessment and management of concussion in sports. *Am Fam Physician.* 1999;60;887-894. Available at: www.aafp.org/afp/990901ap/887.html. Accessed 9/2004.

Nerve Root Assessment—Upper Extremity

Nerve Root	Dermatome	Myotome	Reflex
C4	Top shoulder and neck	Elevate shoulders	—
C5	Lateral upper arm, shoulder	Shoulder abduction	Biceps
C6	Lateral arm, thumb	Elbow flexion/wrist extension	Brachioradialis
C7	Middle finger, posterior middle arm	Elbow extension/wrist flexion	Triceps
C8	Medial hand	Finger flexion	—
T1	Medial elbow	Finger abduction/adduction	—

APPENDIX 11

Nerve Root Assessment—Lower Extremity

Nerve Root	Dermatome	Myotome	Reflex
L1	Anterior upper thigh, lateral hip	Hip flexion	—
L2	Anterior mid thigh	Hip flexion, knee extension	Patella
L3	Lower anterior medial thigh (area of vastus medialis oblique [vmol])	Knee extension	Patella
L4	Anterior/medial leg	Dorsiflexion (heel walking)	Patella
L5	Anterior/lateral leg	Knee flexion, great toe extension	Tibialis posterior
S1	Lateral ankle	Knee flexion, plantar-flexion (toe walking)	Achilles'
S2	Posterior superior lower leg	—	—

Peripheral Nerve Innervations—Upper Extremity

Peripheral Nerve	Sensory Area	Manual Muscle Test
Axillary (C5-6)	Upper deltoid area	Deltoid, teres minor
Musculocutaneous (C5-7)	Anterior and lateral upper arm	Biceps brachii
Radial (C5-T1)	Posterior arm, dorsum of hand	Triceps, wrist extensors
Ulnar (C7-T1)	Anterior/medial forearm, 4th and 5th fingers	Ulnar flexion, flexor digitorum profundus for last two digits
Median (C6-T1)	Anterior/lateral forearm, palmer thumb, 1st, 2nd finger, half of 3rd finger	Thenar eminence, pronators

Musculocutaneous Nerve

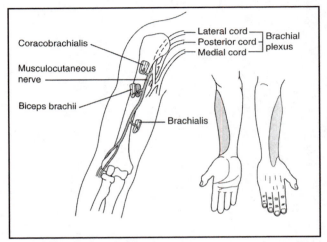

Figure 12-1. Motor and sensory distribution of musculocutaneous nerves (reprinted with permission from Magee D. *Orthopedic Physical Assessment.* 3rd ed. Philadelphia, Pa: WB Saunders; 1997).

Radial and Axillary Nerves

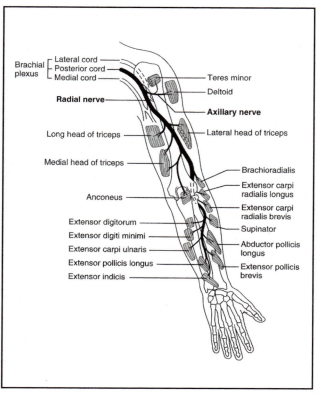

Figure 12-2. Distribution of radial and axillary nerves (reprinted with permission from Magee D. *Orthopedic Physical Assessment.* 3rd ed. Philadelphia, Pa: WB Saunders; 1997).

APPENDIX 13

Peripheral Nerve Innervations—Lower Extremity

Peripheral Nerve	Sensory Area	Manual Muscle Test
Femoral	Medial thigh and leg	Quadriceps
Sciatic (common peroneal and tibial)	Posterior thigh and leg	Hamstrings (tibial)
Obturator	Mid anterior thigh	Adductors
Common peroneal	See deep and superficial peroneal	See deep and superficial peroneal
Deep peroneal	Web space between 1st and 2nd toes	Dorsiflexors
Superficial peroneal	Medial dorsal surface of foot	Evertors
Tibial	Posterior leg	Hamstrings and plantar flexors

Common Peroneal Nerve

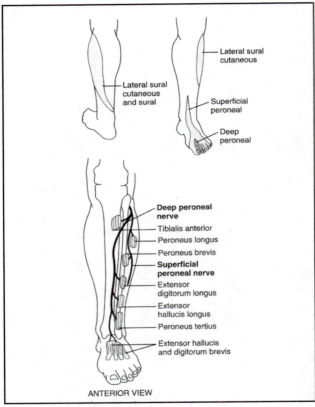

Figure 13-1. Common peroneal nerve (reprinted with permission from Magee D. *Orthopedic Physical Assessment.* 3rd ed. Philadelphia, Pa: WB Saunders; 1997).

Sciatic Nerve

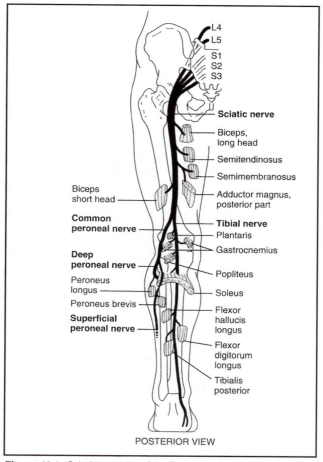

Figure 13-2. Sciatic nerve and its branches (reprinted with permission from Magee D. *Orthopedic Physical Assessment*. 3rd ed. Philadelphia, Pa: WB Saunders; 1997).

Plantar Nerves

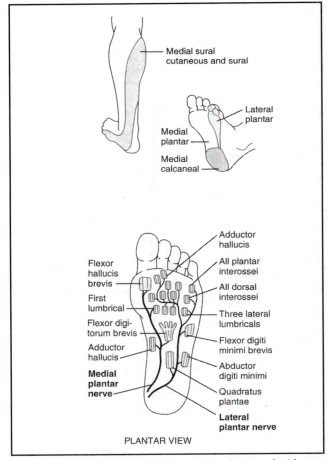

Figure 13-3. Medial and lateral plantar nerves (reprinted with permission from Magee D. *Orthopedic Physical Assessment.* 3rd ed. Philadelphia, Pa: WB Saunders; 1997).

Femoral Nerve

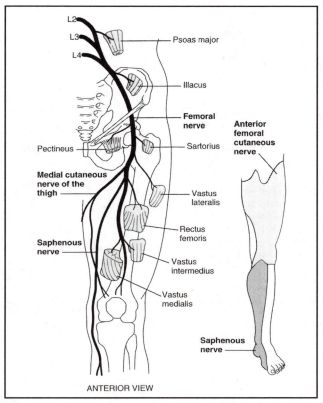

Figure 13-4. Femoral nerve (reprinted with permission from Magee D. *Orthopedic Physical Assessment.* 3rd ed. Philadelphia, Pa: WB Saunders; 1997).

Obturator Nerve

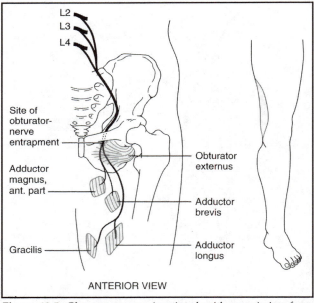

Figure 13-5. Obturator nerve (reprinted with permission from Magee D. *Orthopedic Physical Assessment.* 3rd ed. Philadelphia, Pa: WB Saunders; 1997).

APPENDIX 14

Grades of Pain

I   Patient complains of pain upon palpation

II   Patient complains of pain and winces upon palpation

III   Patient winces and withdraws the injured part upon palpation

IV   Patient will not allow palpation

Appendix 15

End Feel

Normal End Feel

Soft: Created by soft tissue approximation (eg, elbow or knee flexion)

Firm: Created by tissue stretch; stretch may be muscle/tendon, ligament, or capsule (eg, active or passive straight leg raise-hamstring tension)

Hard: Bone on bone (eg, during elbow extension, the olecranon comes into contact with the olecranon fossa)

Abnormal End Feel

Soft: Occurs sooner or later than normal or in a joint that normally has a firm or hard end feel

Firm: Occurs sooner or later than normal or in a joint that normally has a soft or hard end feel

Hard: Occurs sooner or later than normal or in a joint that normally has a firm or soft end feel (feels like a bony block or capsular tightness)

Springy block: Hard end feel with slight spring, occurs sooner than normal end range

Empty: Has no real end feel or pain inhibits reaching end ROM

Causes of Abnormal End Feel

Soft: Inflammation (edema)
Firm: Muscle spasm or shortening, capsular
              shortening
Hard: Fracture, loose bodies, chondromalacia,
              myositis ossificans
Springy block: Meniscal lesion
Empty: Fracture, bursitis, abscess, acute joint
              inflammation, psychogenic origin

APPENDIX 16

Joint Mobility Positioning

A **close-packed position** is a joint position where the bone ends are most congruent and joint surface contact is maximal and compressed.

A **loose (open)-packed position** is a joint position where the joint surfaces are in a position of least congruency and at least part of the capsule is lax. In this position, the joint will exhibit the most laxity. *See* appendix 15.

Rules—Convex on Concave/Concave on Convex:

Concave-Convex Rule: In joint mobilization, the rule related to movement of a concave bone on a convex bone describing accessory motion that is in the same direction as the physiological motion. *See also* convex-concave rule.

Convex-Concave Rule: In joint mobilization, the rule related to movement of a convex bone on a concave bone describing accessory motion that is in the direction opposite the physiological motion. *See also* concave-convex rule.

The Upper Extremity

Joint	Loose-packed	Close-packed
Glenohumeral	55° abd., 30° hor. add.	Max. abd. and ext. rotation
Acromioclavicular	Arm in neutral	90° shoulder abd
Sternoclavicular	Arm in neutral	Max. shoulder elevation
Ulnohumeral	70° elbow flx. 10° sup.	Elbow ext. and sup.
Radiohumeral	Elbow ext. and sup.	90° flx., 5° sup.
Proximal Radioulnar	70° flx., 35° sup.	Ext., 5° sup.
Distal Radioulnar	10° sup.	5° sup.
Radiocarpal	Slight ulnar dev.	Wrist ext. and rad. dev.
Metacarpophalangeal (thumb)	Slight flx.	Opposition
Metacarpophalangeal (four fingers)	Slight flx.	Max. flx.
PIP	10° flx.	Ext.
DIP	30° flx.	Ext.

The Lower Extremity

Joint	Loose-packed	Close-packed
The Hip	30° flx, 30° abd, and ext. rot.	Max ext.
The Knee	25° flx	Ext., ext. rot
Talocrural	10° pf	Max df
Subtalar	10° pf	Max. inv.
Tarsometatarsal	Neutral	Max. sup.
Metatarsophalangeal	Neutral	Max. ext.
Interphalangeal	Slight flx.	Max. ext.

References:

Magee DJ. *Orthopedic Physical Assessment.* 3rd ed. Philadelphia, Pa: WB Saunders; 1997.

Houglum PA. *Therapeutic Exercise for Athletic Injuries.* Champaign, Ill: Human Kinetics; 2001.

Prentice WE. *Therapeutic for Physical Therapists.* 2nd ed. Boston, Mass: McGraw Hill Companies Inc.; 2002.

APPENDIX 17

Special Tests

Shoulder—Ligamentous Tests

Anterior Apprehension Test

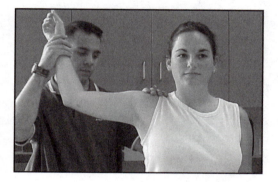

Structure/condition tested: Anterior instability.
Positive sign: Apprehension, pain, feeling of instability.
Test procedure: Patient is positioned with shoulder abducted
(90 degrees), externally rotated, and elbow flexed (90 degrees).
Examiner slowly applies external rotation force.

Jobe's Relocation Test (Fowler's sign)

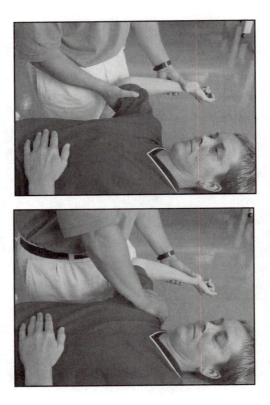

Structure/condition tested: Anterior capsule.
Positive sign: A reduction in pain.
Test procedure: Patient is positioned supine. Examiner performs an anterior apprehension test followed by the same test with anterior stabilization of the glehnohumeral joint (ie, in a posterior direction).

Posterior Apprehension Test

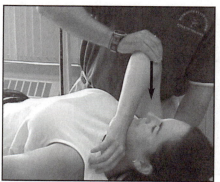

Structure/condition tested: Posterior instability.
Positive sign: Apprehension, pain, or a feeling of instability.
Test procedure: Patient is positioned supine with elbow flexed, shoulder flexed and internally rotated. Examiner applies a posterior force.

Inferior Apprehension Test

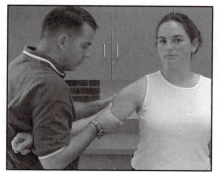

Structure/condition tested: Inferior instability.
Positive sign: Apprehension, pain, sulcus, or instability.
Test procedure: Patient is positioned with shoulder abducted approximately 45 degrees. Examiner applies a slight traction force and a downward (inferior) force.

Sulcus sign

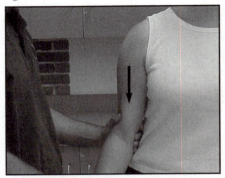

Structure/condition tested: Inferior instability.

Positive sign: Apprehension, pain, a sulcus, or widening of the space.

Test procedure: Patient stands or is positioned seated or supine with arm in relaxed position at side. Examiner applies inferior traction to the humerus.

AC Shear (AC Compression) Test

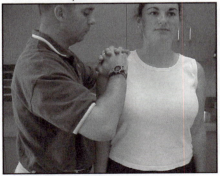

Structure/condition tested: AC joint.

Positive sign: Pain in AC joint or movement of the clavicle.

Test procedure: Patient is seated or standing. Examiner cups hands over the anterior and posterior joint (over clavicle and spine of scapula) and applies compressive force.

O'Brien Test

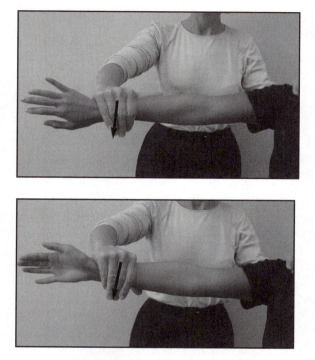

Structure/condition tested: SLAP (superior, labrum, anterior, posterior) lesion.

Positive sign: Pain and/or audible "pop" while internally rotated.

Test procedure: Patient is positioned with shoulder at 90 degrees flexion and internally rotated. Examiner applies a downward force as patient resists. This is repeated with shoulder externally rotated.

Clancy Test

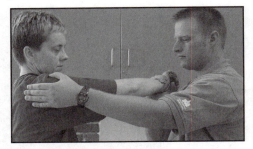

Structure/condition tested: SLAP lesion.
Positive sign: Pain and/or palpable instability.
Test procedure: Test is similar to O'Brien except examiner applies a posterior force to the shoulder joint.

Shoulder—Special Tests

Speeds Test

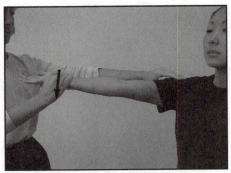

Structure/condition tested: Biceps tendonitis or subluxation.
Positive sign: Pain and weakness in the anterior shoulder indicates biceps tendonitis or tendon subluxation.
Test procedure: Patient is positioned standing or seated with shoulder flexed to 90 degrees, elbow extended, and forearm supinated. Examiner applies a downward (extension) pressure while patient resists with the extended elbow.

Yergason's Test

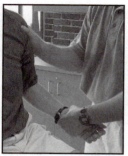

Structure/condition tested: Biceps subluxation.

Positive sign: Pain or an audible "pop" indicates bicep subluxation.

Test procedure: Patient is positioned standing or seated with elbow flexed and forearm supinated. The examiner palpates the bicipital groove and grasps the distal forearm, resisting the patient's attempt to supinate the forearm and laterally rotate the shoulder.

Empty Can Test

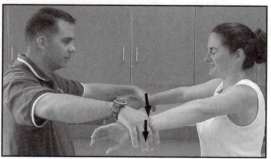

Structure/condition tested: Rotator cuff.

Positive sign: Pain or weakness.

Test procedure: Patient is positioned in shoulder abduction, internal rotation, and slight horizontal flexion. Patient resists examiner's downward force.

Drop Arm Test

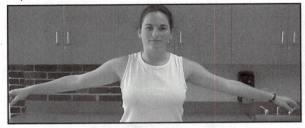

Structure/condition tested: Rotator cuff-supraspinatus.
Positive sign: The inability to control a slow movement.
Test procedure: Patient is positioned in shoulder abduction; have the patient slowly lower the arms.

Allen's Test

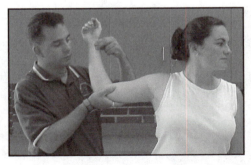

Structure/condition tested: Thoracic outlet syndrome (TOS).
Positive sign: Absent or diminished pulse or radiating pain.
Test procedure: Patient is positioned in shoulder abduction and external rotation with the elbow flexed to 90 degrees. Have the patient rotate the neck to the opposite side. Check pulse.

Adsons Maneuver

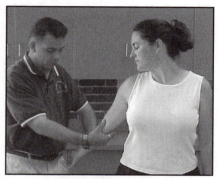

Structure/condition tested: TOS.
Positive sign: Absent or diminished pulse or radiating pain.
Test procedure: Patient is positioned in shoulder extension, external rotation, and neck extension and rotation to the same side. Check pulse.

Halstead Maneuver

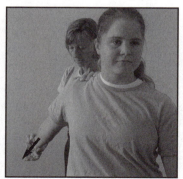

Structure/condition tested: TOS.
Positive sign: Absent or diminished pulse or radiating pain.
Test procedure: Patient is positioned in shoulder extension, external rotation, neck extension, and rotation to the opposite side. Examiner applies a downward traction force to the extremity.

Costoclavicular Test

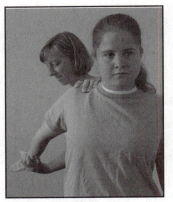

Structure/condition tested: TOS.
Positive sign: Absent or diminished pulse or radiating pain.
Test procedure: Patient maintains a military posture (shoulders retracted). The examiner applies extension and external rotation of the shoulder while checking the pulse.

Roo's Test

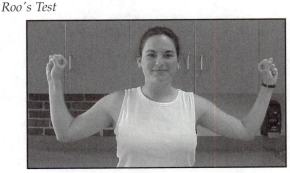

Structure/condition tested: TOS.
Positive sign: Inability to complete the test, absent or diminished pulse, or radiating pain are positive signs.
Test procedure: Patient's shoulders are positioned in active abduction and external rotation with elbows flexed. Patient opens and closes fists for 3 minutes.

Cross-Over Impingement Test

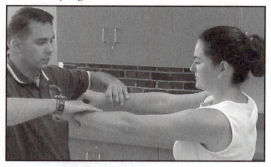

Structure/condition tested: Impingement.
Positive sign: Anterior pain indicates biceps tendon, supraspinatus, or subscapularis impingement. Posterior pain indicates teres minor, infraspinatus, or capsular pathology.
Test procedure: Patient is positioned in shoulder flexion (90 degrees). Examiner resists the patient's shoulder horizontal flexion.

Hawkins-Kennedy Impingement sign

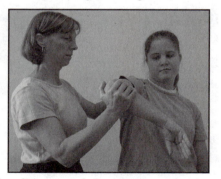

Structure/condition tested: Supra-spinatus impingement or tendinitis.
Positive sign: Pain and weakness.
Test procedure: The patient's shoulder is flexed to 90 degrees and elbow at 90 degrees. The examiner forcibly internally rotates the shoulder with elbow flexed to 90 degrees.

Neer Impingement sign

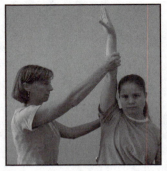

Structure/condition tested: Biceps tendon or supra-spinatus impingement.

Positive sign: Pain and weakness.

Test procedure: Examiner forcibly flexes the shoulder with shoulder internal rotation, elbow extended.

Elbow—Special Tests

Valgus/Varus Stress Test

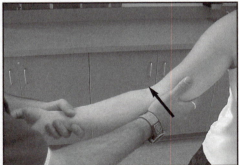

Structure/condition tested: Collateral ligaments.

Positive sign: Joint instability.

Test procedure: Patient's elbow is extended and forearm supinated. Examiner applies a valgus or varus stress to the joint.

Cozen's Test

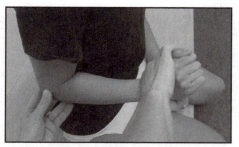

Structure/condition tested: Lateral epicondylitis (extensors).
Positive sign: Pain at lateral epicondyle and/or weakness.
Test procedure: With patient's elbow flexed, examiner palpates the lateral epicondyle and resists the patient's wrist extension/radial deviation.

Mills' Test

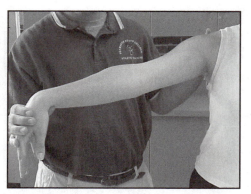

Structure/condition tested: Lateral epicondylitis (extensors).
Positive sign: Pain at the lateral epicondyle.
Test procedure: With the patient's shoulder flexed, elbow extended and pronated, apply passive wrist flexion.

Medial Epicondylitis Test

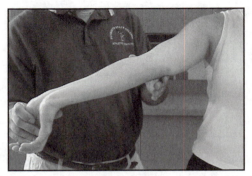

Structure/condition tested: Medial epicondylitis (flexors).
Positive sign: Pain at the medial epicondyle.
Test procedure: Same as Mills' test but the examiner applies passive wrist extension with patient forearm supinated.

Elbow Flexion Test

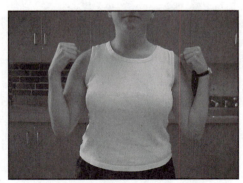

Structure/condition tested: Ulnar nerve entrapment.
Positive sign: Pain or numbness/tingling in the ulnar nerve distribution.
Test procedure: Patient is positioned in elbow flexion and asked to hold the position for 1 minute.

Whartenberg's sign

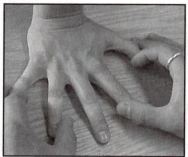

Structure/condition tested: Ulnar nerve neuropathy.
Positive sign: Inability to return 5th finger to the hand.
Test procedure: Patient's hand is positioned flat on a table. Examiner passively abducts the patient's fingers. The patient is then instructed to adduct the little finger toward the other fingers.

Pronator Teres Syndrome

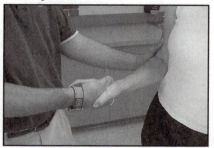

Structure/condition tested: Median nerve entrapment.
Positive sign: Pain and/or numbness/tingling in median nerve distribution or weakness as compared to contrallateral side.
Test procedure: Patient is positioned seated or standing with elbow flexed approximately 70-90 degrees with forearm in neutral position. Examiner stabilizes patient's arm at the elbow with one hand. Patient and examiner may grasp hands as in a handshake, or examiner may stabilize forearm above the wrist. Examiner resists patient's attempt at pronation.

Tinel's sign

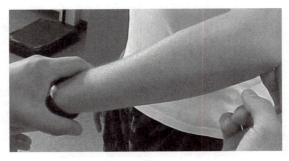

Structure/condition tested: Ulnar nerve injury.
Positive sign: Pain and/or tingling in ulnar nerve distribution.
Test procedure: Examiner taps over the patient's ulnar nerve.

Hand/Wrist—Special Tests

Phalen's Test

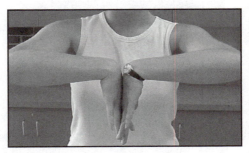

Structure/condition tested: Carpal tunnel syndrome.
Positive sign: Pain and/or paresthesia of the thumb and first two fingers.
Test procedure: Patient places the dorsal surface of the hands together and pushes wrists into flexion. This position is held for 1 minute.

Murphy's sign

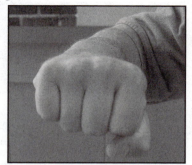

Structure/condition tested: Lunate dislocation.
Positive sign: The head of the 3rd metacarpal is level with the heads of the 2nd and 4th metacarpals.
Test procedure: Patient is asked to make a fist.

Watson's Test (Scaphoid Shift Test)

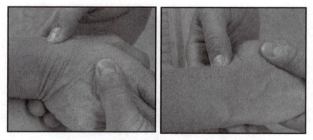

Structure/condition tested: Scaphoid/lunate instability.
Positive sign: Subluxation of the scaphoid dorsally above the edge of the radius and the patient complains of pain.
Test procedure: The patient is positioned seated with the arm pronated and resting on the thigh or on a table. The examiner stabilizes the distal end of the scaphoid and passively moves the wrist into full ulnar deviation and slight extension. The examiner then passively moves the joint into radial deviation and slight flexion.

Tinel's sign

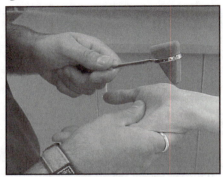

Structure/condition tested: Median/ulnar nerve.
Positive sign: Pain and/or paresthesia along nerve distribution.
Test procedure: Examiner taps over the median (in the carpal tunnel) or ulnar nerve (in the tunnel of Guyon) as they cross the palmer surface of the wrist.

Finkelstein's Test

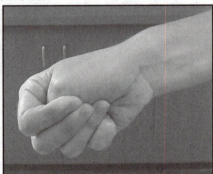

Structure/condition tested: De Quervain's disease.
Positive sign: Pain along the lateral aspect of the wrist.
Test procedure: Patient places the thumb inside the closed fist and performs wrist ulnar deviation or the examiner performs passive ulnar deviation.

Thumb Hyperextension Test

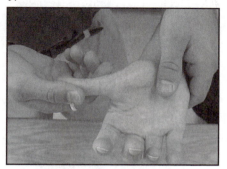

Structure/condition tested: Volar plate.
Positive sign: Abnormal joint movement/instability and/or pain.
Test procedure: Examiner applies hyperextension force to the metacarpophalangeal (MCP) joint to assess ligamentous integrity.

Bunnel/Littler Test

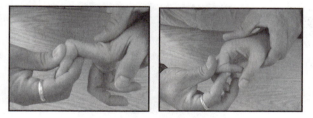

Structure/condition tested: PIP contracture.
Positive sign: Limited range with MCP extended indicates tight intrinsics; limited range with MCP flexed indicates capsular tightness.
Test procedure: Assess flexion PROM of the PIP with the MCP slightly extended. Compare to PROM when MCP is slightly flexed.

Neck—Ligamentous Tests

Compression Test

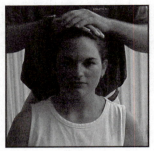

Structure/condition tested: Nerve root compression.
Positive sign: Neck pain or radicular pain.
Test procedure: Patient is seated with head in neutral position. Examiner applies compression/axial load.

Foraminal Compression Test (Spurling's Test)

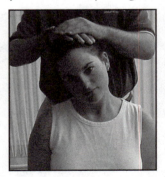

Structure/condition tested: Nerve root compression, foraminal compression.
Positive sign: Neck pain or radicular pain.
Test procedure: Patient is seated with neck laterally flexed to one side. Examiner applies compression/axial load.

Jackson Compression Test

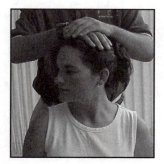

Structure/condition tested: Nerve root compression.
Positive sign: Neck pain or radicular pain.
Test procedure: Patient is seated with neck rotated to one side. Examiner applies compression/axial load.

Maximum Cervical Compression Test

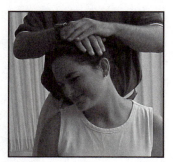

Structure/condition tested: Nerve root compression.
Positive sign: Neck pain or radicular pain.
Test procedure: Patient is seated with neck laterally flexed and rotated to one side. Examiner applies compression/axial load.

Distraction Test

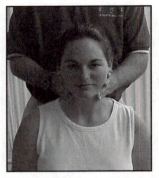

Structure/condition tested: Nerve root compression.
Positive sign: The relief of symptoms.
Test procedure: Patient is seated with neck in neutral position. Examiner applies distraction to the head/neck.

Shoulder Depression Test

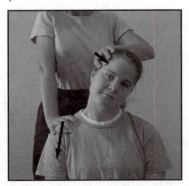

Structure/condition tested: Brachial plexus traction injury and positive pain/radiculopathy along dermatome.
Positive sign: Neck pain and especially radicular pain.
Test procedure: Patient is seated with neck laterally flexed to one side. Examiner depresses patient's opposite shoulder.

Spine—Special Tests

Lasegues

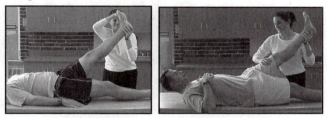

Structure/condition tested: Nerve root involvement.

Positive sign: Back pain and/or radicular pain of the *involved* limb that returns on dorsiflexion or active neck flexion.

Test procedure: Patient is positioned supine. Examiner performs a passive straight leg raise (SLR) of the affected leg to the point of pain. Examiner then lowers the leg until the patient's pain is gone. Examiner passively dorsiflexes the ankle. If pain does not return, ask patient to actively flex neck.

Well Straight Leg Raise (SLR) Test

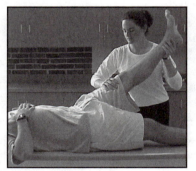

Structure/condition tested: Nerve root involvement.

Positive sign: Back pain and/or radicular pain of the *involved* limb.

Test procedure: Patient is positioned supine. Examiner performs a passive SLR of the *uninvolved* limb.

Kernig (Brudzinski) sign

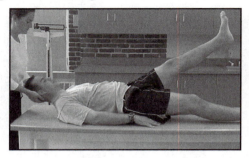

Structure/condition tested: Nerve root involvement.
Positive sign: Back pain and/or radicular pain of the involved limb.
Test procedure: Similar to Lasegues, except patient performs active SLR of involved limb. Examiner provides passive neck flexion for the patient.

Milgrams Test

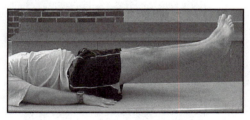

Structure/condition tested: Nerve root involvement.
Positive sign: The inability to perform the test or the production of pain.
Test procedure: Patient is positioned supine. Patient performs a bilateral SLR and holds this position for 30 seconds.

Valsalva's Maneuver

Structure/condition tested: Nerve root involvement
Positive sign: Back pain and radicular pain
Test procedure: Patient is asked to bear down (alternate method is to have patient blow into closed fist)

Bowstring Test (Cram/Popliteal Pressure Test)

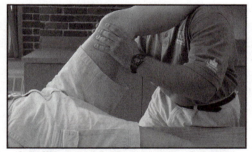

Structure/condition tested: Nerve root involvement.
Positive sign: Pain indicates sciatic nerve compression or tension.
Test procedure: Patient is positioned supine. The examiner performs a passive SLR to the point of pain and then allows knee flexion until pain is relieved. The examiner then applies pressure to the popliteal space.

Facet Joint Test

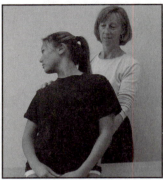

Structure/condition tested: Facet joints.
Positive sign: Back pain is reproduced.
Test procedure: The standing patient extends, laterally flexes, and rotates trunk toward the painful side.

Hoover Test (Malingering Test)

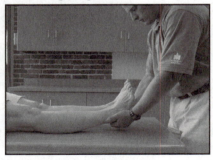

Structure/condition tested: Malingering.
Positive sign: If the patient cannot raise the leg and the examiner does not feel pressure under the patient's uninvolved heel, the patient may be malingering.
Test procedure: The patient is positioned supine. The examiner places one hand under each calcaneus between the patient and the table. The patient is asked to perform a straight leg raise.

Sacroiliac Joint

FABER Test (Patrick's Test)

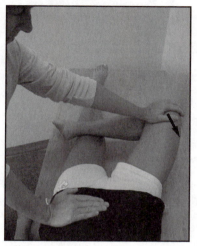

Structure/condition tested: Sacroiliac dysfunction, hip internal rotation contracture.

Positive sign: The inability to move the thigh parallel to the table or the production of sacroiliac pain.

Test procedure: Flexion, abduction, external rotation. Patient is positioned supine with one ankle crossed over the opposite knee. Examiner applies pressure to the ASIS and knee of the crossed leg.

Yeoman's Test

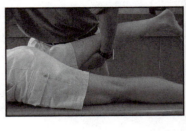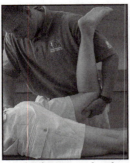

Structure/condition tested: Sacroiliac dysfunction, lumbar involvement, femoral nerve stretch.

Positive sign: Pain in the low back (during all movements) indicates lumbar involvement; pain in the sacroiliac area (during all movements) indicates anterior sacroiliac ligament injury, femoral nerve stretch; and pain in the anterior hip/thigh area (during all movements) indicates femoral nerve stretch.

Test procedure: Patient is positioned prone. Examiner passively extends each hip first with the knee extended and then with knee flexed.

Gapping Test

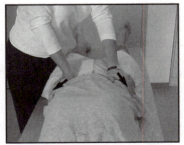

Structure/condition tested: Sacroiliac dysfunction.

Positive sign: Pain in the sacroiliac joint or radicular pain.

Test procedure: Patient is positioned supine. Examiner applies a "down and out" pressure to the ASIS.

Squish Test

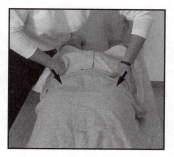

Structure/condition tested: Sacroiliac dysfunction.
Positive sign: Pain in the sacroiliac joint or radicular pain.
Test procedure: Same as the gapping test but the examiner applies pressure "down and in" .

Sacral Apex Test

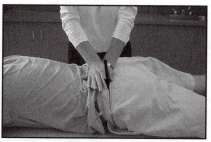

Structure/condition tested: Sacroiliac dysfunction.
Positive sign: Pain in the sacroiliac joint or radicular pain.
Test procedure: Patient is positioned prone. Examiner applies force straight down on the sacrum

Gaenslin's Test

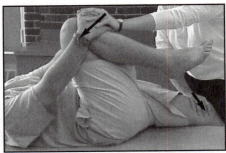

Structure/condition tested: Sacroiliac dysfunction.
Positive sign: Pain in the sacroiliac joint or radicular pain.
Test procedure: Patient is positioned supine near the edge of the examination table. The patient's limb is positioned over the edge of the table so as to allow passive hip extension and knee flexion. The opposite knee and hip are flexed and pressure is applied to both limbs.

Hip—Special Tests

Sign of the Buttocks

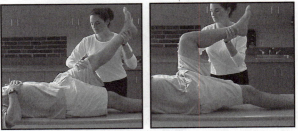

Structure/condition tested: Trochanteric bursitis, tumor.
Positive sign: No increase in hip flexion ROM is a positive sign for bursitis, tumor, or other hip joint pathology.
Test procedure: Patient is positioned supine. Examiner performs a passive SLR to the point of pain or the early end of range of motion. Examiner then attempts further hip flexion with knee flexed.

Ely's Test

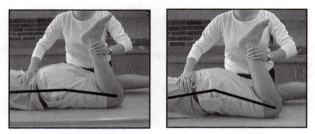

Structure/condition tested: Rectus femoris contracture.
Positive sign: Hip is unable to stay flat on table, an indication of tight rectus femoris muscle.
Test procedure: Patient is positioned prone with the knee flexed. The examiner applies further knee flexion

Kendall Test

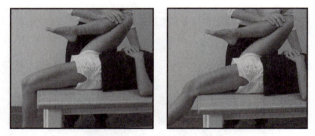

Structure/condition tested: Rectus femoris contracture.
Positive sign: Knee extends, indicating a tight rectus femoris.
Test procedure: Patient is positioned supine near the end of the table with hip extended, knee flexed, and lower leg hanging off the edge of the table. The examiner passively applies hip and knee flexion to the contralateral limb.

Thomas Test

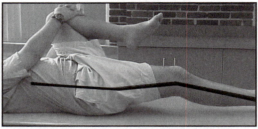

Structure/condition tested: Hip flexor contracture.
Positive sign: Hip flexes as the pelvis is "tilted" anteriorly causing the knee of test leg to flex, indicating tight hip flexors.
Test procedure: Similar to Kendall Test except the patient is positioned supine on the table with both hips and knees extended. The examiner passively applies hip and knee flexion to the uninvolved limb.

Trendelenburg's Test

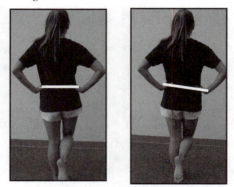

Structure/condition tested: Gluteus medius weakness.
Positive sign: Inability to maintain a level pelvis is positive for weak gluteus medius.
Test procedure: Examiner is positioned behind the patient. Patient is asked to stand on the affected limb.

Ober's Test

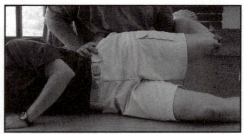

Structure/condition tested: Tensor fascia contracture.
Positive sign: Adduction ROM is limited.
Test procedure: Patient is positioned side lying with the unaffected limb down. Examiner abducts and extends the hip with the knee in flexion. The examiner then passively lowers the hip into adduction while maintaining hip extension and knee flexion.

Knee—Ligamentous Tests

Anterior Draw sign

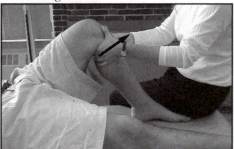

Structure/condition tested: Anteromedial bundle of the anterior cruciate ligament.
Positive sign: Joint instability or laxity.
Test procedure: Patient is positioned supine with knee flexed to 90 degrees. Examiner grasps the tibia just distal to the knee joint and applies an anterior force, assessing the integrity of the anterior cruciate ligament.

Slocum

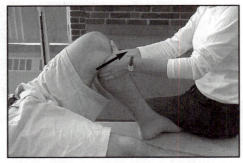

Structure/condition tested: Anterior cruciate ligament.
Positive sign: Joint instability or laxity.
Test procedure: A variation on the anterior draw sign in which the tibia is rotated internally and externally prior to the application of the anterior draw.

Lachman's Test

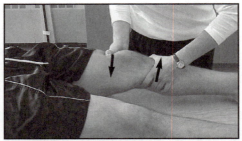

Structure/condition tested: Posterolateral bundle of the anterior cruciate ligament.
Positive sign: Joint instability or laxity.
Test procedure: Patient is positioned supine. Examiner grasps the patient's leg just above and below the knee and positions the knee in slight flexion (approximately 10 degrees to 15 degrees). While stabilizing the thigh, the examiner applies an anterior force to the tibia.

Pivot Shift Test

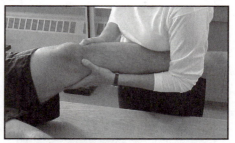

Structure/condition tested: Anterior cruciate ligament.
Positive sign: As the knee is flexed to approximately 30 degrees to 40 degrees, the tibia will shift posteriorly back into position.
Test procedure: Patient is positioned supine. Examiner grasps the patient's leg on either side of the knee and positions the knee in slight flexion. The examiner applies a valgus force and internal tibial rotation while further flexing the knee.

Posterior Draw sign

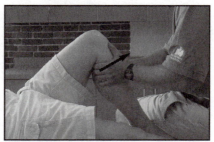

Structure/condition tested: Posterior cruciate ligament.
Positive sign: Joint instability or laxity.
Test procedure: Patient is positioned supine with knee flexed to 90 degrees. Examiner grasps the tibia just distal to the knee joint and applies a posterior force over the tibial tubercle to stress the posterior cruciate ligament.

Posterior Sag Test (Profile Test)

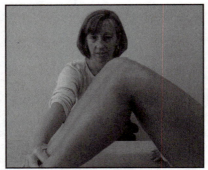

Structure/condition tested: Posterior cruciate ligament.
Positive sign: Posterior sag.
Test procedure: Patient is positioned supine with knee flexed to 90 degrees. Examiner stands to the side and observes the tibial tubercle for a posterior sag as compared to the opposite limb.

Godfrey's Test (Godfrey's 90-90 test)

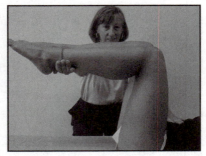

Structure/condition tested: Posterior cruciate ligament.
Positive sign: Posterior sag.
Test procedure: With the patient positioned supine with the hips and knees at 90 degrees, observe the tibial tubercle for a posterior sag in comparison to the opposite limb.

Valgus Stress

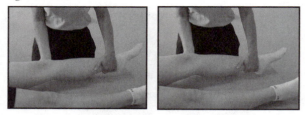

Structure/condition tested: Medial collateral ligament/ medial capsule.

Positive sign: Joint instability or laxity.

Test procedure: The patient is positioned supine. The examiner grasps the patient's lower leg and applies a valgus force at the knee joint line to stress the medial collateral and capsular ligaments. This test is performed with knee fully extended and flexed to 20 degrees.

Varus Stress Test

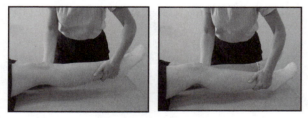

Structure/condition tested: Lateral collateral ligament/lateral capsule.

Positive sign: Joint instability or laxity.

Test procedure: The patient is positioned supine. The examiner grasps the patient's lower leg and applies a varus force at the knee joint line to stress the lateral collateral and capsular ligaments. This test is performed with knee fully extended and flexed to 20 degrees.

Knee—Meniscal Tests

Bounce Home Test

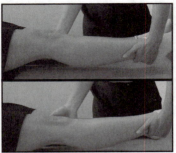

Structure/condition tested: Meniscus.

Positive sign: ROM that is limited or end range that is springy, a meniscal lesion could be the cause.

Test procedure: The patient is positioned supine with the knee slightly flexed. The examiner allows the knee to drop slowly into extension.

Apley's Compression Test

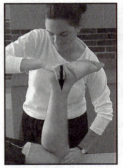

Structure/condition tested: Meniscus.

Positive sign: Pain, locking, or catching are positive signs for meniscal tear.

Test procedure: The patient is positioned prone with the knee flexed to 90 degrees. The examiner grasps the patient's foot and applies a longitudinal force along the shaft of the tibia and rotates the tibia internally and externally.

Apley's Distraction Test

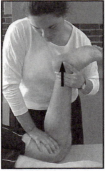

Structure/condition tested: Meniscus.

Positive sign: A relief of pain indicates meniscal tear.

Test procedure: Positioning is the same as for Apley's compression test except that a distraction force is applied by grasping the patient's ankle and stabilizing the thigh.

McMurray Test

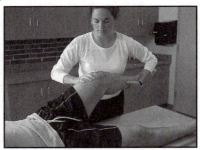

Structure/condition tested: Meniscus.

Positive sign: Pain, locking, or catching are positive signs for meniscal tear.

Test procedure: The patient is positioned supine. The examiner grasps the patient's leg just above the knee and just proximal to the ankle. The examiner applies a valgus and varus force combining internal and external tibial rotation while flexing and extending the knee.

Knee and Leg—Other Special Tests

Homan's Sign

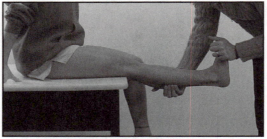

Structure/condition tested: Deep vein thrombophlebitis.

Positive sign: Pain in calf when stretch is applied; loss of or diminished dorsal pedal pulse; examiner may observe swelling or palor.

Test procedure: The patient is positioned supine. Examiner extends knee and passively dorsiflexes foot.

Noble Compression Test

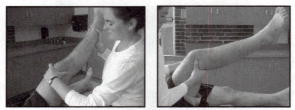

Structure/condition tested: Iliotibial band friction syndrome as the iliotibial band crosses over the lateral femoral condyle at the knee.

Positive sign: Pain as the iliotibial band crosses over the lateral epicondyle is a positive sign.

Test procedure: Patient is positioned supine. The examiner palpates the lateral femoral epicondyle while flexing and extending the patient's knee. An alternate method is to have the patient perform active knee extension.

Patella Apprehension Test

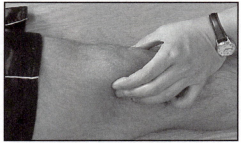

Structure/condition tested: Patella subluxation.
Positive sign: Apprehension upon contraction.
Test procedure: Patient is positioned supine. With knee extended and patient relaxed, the examiner applies a gentle lateral force to the patella.

Patella Tracking Test

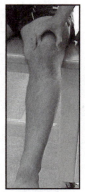

Structure/condition tested: Patella tracking dysfunction.
Positive sign: Abnormal tracking.
Test procedure: With the patient seated at the edge of the table, knee at 90 degrees, the examiner places the hand over the lateral edges of the patella. The patient slowly extends and flexes the knee through a full range of motion. Patella should move superiorly and slightly laterally in a smooth coordinated motion.

Crunch/Grind Test

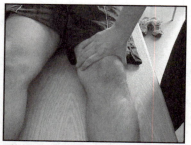

Structure/condition tested: Chondromalacia.
Positive sign: Pain and a crunching or grinding sensation.
Test procedure: The patient is positioned supine with the knee extended and leg relaxed. The examiner applies a stabilizing force just proximal to the patella. The patient then slowly contracts the quadriceps. Warning—this test is painful even to asymptomatic individuals. Apply cautiously.

Foot/Ankle—Ligamentous Tests

Anterior Draw Test

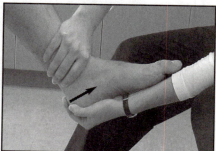

Structure/condition tested: Anterior talofibular, deltoid, anterior tibiofibular.
Positive sign: Joint laxity and/or pain.
Test procedure: The patient is seated with knee flexed to 90 degrees. The examiner stabilizes the tibia with one hand and grasps the calcaneus and "draws" (pulls) forward to assess the integrity of the ligaments.

Anterior Draw Test 2

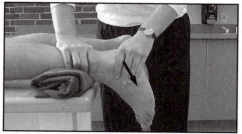

Structure/condition tested: Anterior talofibular, deltoid, anterior tibiofibular.

Positive sign: Joint laxity and/or pain.

Test procedure: The patient is positioned prone with the foot hanging off the edge of the table, with padding under the distal tibia. The examiner applies a downward (anterior) pressure to the calcaneus to assess the integrity of the ligaments.

Talar Tilt

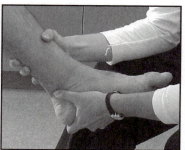

Structure/condition tested: Inversion-neutral-calcaneofibular, dorsi-post talofibular, plantar-anterior talofibular, eversion-deltoid.

Positive sign: Joint laxity.

Test procedure: The patient is seated with the knee flexed to 90 degrees. The examiner stabilizes the tibia, grasps the calcaneus, and applies inversion and eversion stresses. It is performed in neutral, dorsiflexion, and plantar flexion.

Kleiger Test (also called External Rotation Test)

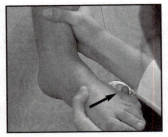

Structure/condition tested: Deltoid, anterior tibiofibular.
Positive sign: Joint laxity.
Test procedure: The patient is seated with the knee flexed to 90 degrees and ankle at 90 degrees. The examiner stabilizes the tibia, grasps the foot, and applies a lateral rotation force.

Midtarsal Test

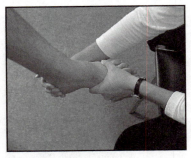

Structure/condition tested: Midtarsal ligaments.
Positive sign: Pain or abnormal motion.
Test procedure: The patient is seated with the knee flexed to 90 degrees. The examiner stabilizes the calcaneus, grasps the midfoot (approximately over the first metatarsophalangeal joint), and applies a torsion (twisting motion) to stress the midtarsal ligaments.

Foot/Ankle—Special Tests

Thompson's Test

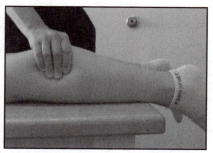

Structure/condition tested: Achilles' tendon rupture.
Positive sign: No plantar flexion is a sign of a ruptured Achilles' tendon.
Test procedure: The patient is positioned prone with knee extended. The examiner grasps the triceps surae and squeezes.

Bump/Tap Test

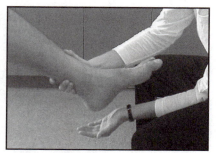

Structure/condition tested: Fibular and tibular fracture.
Positive sign: Pain at site of potential fracture.
Test procedure: The examiner creates a "vibration" along the long axis of the lower leg by "bumping/tapping" the calcaneus.

Squeeze (Compression) Test

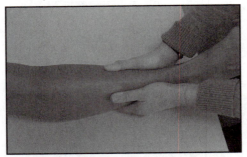

Structure/condition tested: Syndesmosis injury, stress fracture.

Positive sign: Pain upon compression.

Test procedure: Use when fracture and compartment syndrome have been ruled out. The patient is positioned supine. The examiner grasps the middle of the lower leg and "squeezes" the tibia and fibula together.

Toe Distract Test

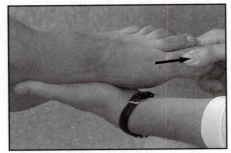

Structure/condition tested: Ligament sprain.

Positive sign: Sprain.

Test procedure: The examiner stabilizes the proximal segment and applies a traction force to the distal segment.

Toe Tap Test

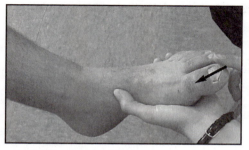

Structure/condition tested: Fracture.
Positive sign: Contusion, fracture.
Test procedure: The examiner applies a light tap to the long axis of the toe.

APPENDIX 18

*Pharmacology**

Reprinted with permission from Jacobs K. *Quick Reference Dictionary for Occupational Therapy.* 2nd ed. Thorofare, NJ: SLACK Incorporated; 1999.

Alcohol Withdrawal
Librium
ReVia
Valium

Alzheimer's Disease
Aricept
Cognex

Angina
Adalat
Inderal
Isoptin
Procardia

Anxiety Disorders
Benzodiazepines:
Ativan
Klonopin
Valium
Xanax
Beta-Blockers:
Inderal
Miscellaneous:
BuSpar

Arthritis
Actron
Advil
Anaprox
Ansaid
Bextra
Celebrex
Daypro
Feldene
Indocin
Lodine
Motrin
Naprosyn
Pediapred
Relafen
Rufen
Toradol
Viox

Asthma
Accolate
Advair
Albuterol
Alupent
AeroBid

*Note: The following is a list of brand name and generic drugs. Please consult each drug's literature for further information. Mention of specific products is not intended as an endorsement by the author or publisher.

Azmacort
Brethine
Intal
Lufyllin
Medrol
Nasacort
Provental
Proventil
Theo-Dur
Ventolin

**Attention Deficit
Hyperactivity
Disorder**
Adderall
Cylert
Dexedrine
Ritalin

Cancer
Arimidex
Cisplatin
Cytoxan
Deltasone
Efudex
Estrace
Estraderm
Medrol
Methotrexate
Orasone
Pediapred
Premarin
Tamoxifen
Taxol

Depression
*Tricyclic
Antidepressants:*
Aventyl
Elavil
Norpramin
Pamelor
Sinequan
Tofranil
*Serotonin Uptake
Inhibitors:*
Paxil
Prozac
Zoloft
*Monoamine Oxidase
(MAO) Inhibitors:*
Lithium
Nardil
Parnate
Miscellaneous:
Desyrel
Effexor
Lithium
Serzone
Vivactil
Wellbutrin

Fluid Retention
Bumex
Diamox
Diuril
Dyazide
Esidrix
Lasix
Lozol

Maxzide
Thalitone

Headache, Cluster
Calan
Depakote
Lithium
Sansert

Headache, Migraine
Amerge
Cafergot
Imitrex
Inderal
Maxalt
Midrin
Nadolol
Wygesic
Zomig

Headache, Tension
Anolor
Esgic
Fioricet
Fiorinal
Fiorinal with Codeine

Heart Attack
Atenolol
Captopril
Inderal
Lopressor
Prinivil
Tenormin
Zestril

High Blood Pressure
Accupril
Adalat
Aldomet
Altace
Calan
Catapres
Lasix
Lopressor
Lotrel
Moduretic
Norvasc
Procardia

Infection, HIV
Crixivan
Epivir
Hivid
Invirase
Norvir
Retrovir
Videx
Viramune
Zerit

**Infections, Lower
Respiratory Tract**
Amoxil
Augmentin
Biaxin
Ceclor
Ceftin
E-Mycin
Flagyl
Ilotycin

Keflex
Pen-Vee K
Tetracycline
Zithromax

Infections, Upper Respiratory Tract
Amoxicillin with Clavulanate
Augmentin
Bactrin
Ceclor
Ceftin
E-Mycin
Flagyl
Keflex
Tetracycline

Inflammatory Diseases
Anaprox
Celebrex
Decadron Tablets
Deltasone
Ibuprofen
Medrol
Naproxen Sodium
Orasone
Pediapred
Viox

Insomnia
Ambien
Dalmane
Desyrel
Doral
Halcion

ProSom
Restoril

Muscle Relaxants
Flexeril
Norflex
Norgesic
Robaxin
Skelaxin
Soma
Valium

Neuropathy
Amatriptolene
Neurontin

Obsessive-Compulsive Disorder
Anafranil
Luvox
Paxil
Prozac

Osteoporosis
Calcimar
Estrace
Estraderm
Fosamax
Miacalcin
Ogen
Premarin

Paget's Disease
Alendronate Sodium
Calcimar
Fosamax
Miacalcin

Pain

Acetaminophen
Anaprox
Ansaid
Cataflam
Clinoril
Darvocet-N
Darvon
Demerol
Ecotrin
Empirin with
   Codeine
Lorcet
Motrin
Naprosyn
Panadol
Talwin
Toradol
Voltaren

Parkinson's Disease

Artane
Benadryl
Cogentin
Eldepryl
Mirapex
Parlodel
Permax
Requip
Sinemet CR
Symmetrel
TaSmar

Sexually Transmitted Diseases

Acyclovir
Amoxil

Ceftin
Doryx
E-Mycin
Flagyl
Floxin
Minocin
Omnipen
Zonirax

Schizophrenia

Antipsychotics:
Haldol
Mellaril
Risperdal
Stelazine
Thorazine

Seizure Disorders

Cerebyx
Depakote
Dilantin
Lamictal
Neurotonin
Phenobarbital
Tegretol

Ulcers, Peptic

Axid
Biaxin
Carafate
Prilosec
Tagamet
Zantac

Resources

PDR Family Guide to Prescription Drugs. 6th ed. New York, NY: Three Rivers Press; 1998.

Physicians' Desk Reference. 52nd ed. Montvale, NJ: Medical Economics; 1999.

APPENDIX 19

NATA Membership Standards and Code of Ethics*

I. MEMBERSHIP STANDARDS

In accepting membership in NATA, an applicant agrees that:

A. He or she will comply with the Charter, by-laws, policies, rules, and standards of NATA and the laws and regulations governing NATA. The applicant also agrees to bear the burden for demonstrating and maintaining compliance with these provisions at all times.

B. The cards and logos of NATA, the name "National Athletic Trainers' Association, Inc.," the term "NATA," the terms "ATC" and "CAT," and abbreviations relating thereto are all exclusive property of the NATA and may not be used in any way without the express written consent of NATA.

C. The individual shall immediately relinquish, refrain from using and correct at the individual's expense any outdated or other inaccurate use of any NATA card, logo, mark, and emblem and of the NATA name and related abbreviations, in case of suspension, limitation, or cancellation by, or resignation from NATA, or as otherwise requested by NATA.

D. If the individual refuses to relinquish immediately, refrain from using and correct at his or her expense any misuse or misleading use of any of the above items when requested, the individual agrees that NATA shall be entitled to obtain injunctive relief, damages, costs and attorney's fees incurred in obtaining any such or other relief.

---

*Note: At the time of publication the NATA was in the process of revising this document. Please refer to www.nata.org for the latest version.

II. Eligibility for Membership

A. No individual is eligible for membership unless he or she agrees to comply, and, when a member, is in compliance with all NATA Charter provisions, By-laws, policies, rules, standards, and other governing laws and regulations. NATA may take appropriate action with respect to members' violations of these Charter provisions, By-laws, policies, rules, standards and other governing laws and regulations.

B. The individual must truthfully complete and sign an application in the form provided by NATA and shall provide additional information as requested. The individual must notify NATA of any change in address, telephone number, and any other facts bearing on eligibility or membership within thirty (30) days of such occurrence.

C. An individual convicted of a felony directly related to public health, athletic care, or education shall be ineligible to apply for membership for a period of one year from the exhaustion of appeals, completion of sentence, or completion of parole, whichever is later. Convictions of this nature include but are not limited to felonies involving: rape; sexual abuse of an athlete or child; actual or threatened use of a weapon or violence; the prohibited sale or distribution of a controlled substance, or its possession with the intent to distribute; or use of position of athletic trainer improperly (i) to influence or attempt to influence the outcome or score of an athletic event or (ii) in connection with any gambling activity.

III. MEMBERSHIP SANCTIONS AND PROCEDURES

A. *Grounds for Sanctions*

When a person becomes a member of NATA, he or she assumes certain obligations and responsibilities. A member is responsible for dues as provided and specified by the By-laws or other governing provisions. A member may be subject to one or more of the sanctions set forth in Section III G, below, if his or her conduct falls within one of the following categories:

1. Misstatement of a material fact or failure to state a material fact in an application for membership, or in any other manner obtaining or attempting to obtain NATA membership by fraud or deception;

2. Knowingly assisting another to obtain or attempt to obtain NATA membership by false statement, fraud or deception;

3. Misrepresentation of NATA membership status;

4. Misrepresentation of NATA certification status, or other professional qualification or credentials;

5. The conviction of, plea of guilty or plea of nolo contendere to a felony which is directly related to public health or athletic care or education. This includes but is not limited to a felony involving: rape; sexual abuse of an athlete or child; actual or threatened use of a weapon or violence; the prohibited sale or distribution of a controlled substance, or its possession with the intent to distribute; or use of position of athletic trainer improperly (i) to influence or attempt to influence the outcome or score of an athletic event or (ii) in connection with any gambling activity.

6. Serious or repeated violations of the NATA's Charter, By-laws, Code of Ethics, policies, rules or standards.

B. Panels

1. With general oversight from the NATA Board of Directors, the NATA Ethics Committee, by majority vote, shall select persons who are NATA members to form (i) an Investigative Panel of NATA members, (ii) a Fact-Finding Panel of NATA members, and (iii) an Appellate Panel of NATA members, to address alleged violations of the standards set forth in Sections III A(1)-(6), above. The majority of each of these panels shall consist of Ethics Committee members, and a majority of each of the Presiding Panels selected to handle individual cases shall, if possible, be Ethics Committee members. The Ethics Committee shall attempt to staff Presiding Panels with members from (a) a variety of practice settings, (b) geographically diverse locations, and (c) diverse backgrounds and levels of experience.

2. The terms of the members of each of the three Panels shall run for two years and may be renewed.

3. A majority of the members of each Panel shall annually elect the Chair of that Panel.

4. In every individual case, three members of the Investigative Panel shall carry out the requisite investigative function; three members of the Fact-Finding Panel shall carry out the requisite hearing function; and three members of the Appellate Panel (one Ethics Committee member, one at-large member, and one director from the Board) shall carry out the requisite appellate function. The Chair of each Panel shall determine the identity of the Presiding Panel members assigned to carry out such functions in each case, after due consideration is given to fairness, efficiency, and convenience to all concerned.

5. In every individual case, NATA shall, upon written request from the Investigative or Fact-Finding Panels, provide to said Panels all information in the custody of NATA related to the NATA applicant or member in

question. Each NATA applicant or member in question shall release, discharge, and exonerate NATA, its officers, directors, employees, committee members, and agents furnishing said information, from any and all liability of any nature and kind arising out of or relating to the furnishing of said information.

6. No NATA member shall serve concurrently on more than one of the three Panels.

7. No NATA member shall serve on more than one Presiding Panel in the same case.

8. No member of any of the three Panels shall participate in any case where his or her impartiality or the presence of an actual, potential or apparent conflict of interest might reasonably be questioned.

9. When a vacancy occurs on one of the three Panels, the Ethics Committee by majority vote shall promptly elect a replacement from among the NATA membership.

C.   *Reporting of Violations*

NATA members who have information with regard to allegations raising issues under Sections III A(1)-(6), above, and wishing to supply such information to NATA, shall supply this information, with as much specificity and documentation as possible, to NATA's Executive Director or Chair of the Ethics Committee. If an NATA member supplies information to only one of these two individuals, the individual receiving the information shall notify the other, and supply copies of any letters or other documents received. If an NATA member, or someone who is not an NATA member, supplies information concerning a possible violation of NATA standards to an NATA member other than the Executive Director or the Ethics Committee Chair, that member may forward the information to the Executive Director or Ethics Committee Chair, or encourage the individual or individuals supplying the information to do so.

Information need not be supplied in writing, and the reporting NATA member need not identify him or herself. However, NATA's Executive Director and Ethics Committee Chair will not forward information that is too vague, information that cannot be substantiated without the assistance of the reporting person, or information where, in the opinion of the NATA Executive Director and Ethics Chair, there is no need for anonymity for the reporting individual.

A member may report information on the condition that the member's name or certain other facts be kept confidential.

NATA may proceed with an investigation subject to such a condition; however, NATA must inform the reporting member that at some point in the investigation NATA may determine that it cannot proceed further without disclosing some of the confidential information, either to the applicant or member under investigation or to some other party. A reporting member, upon receiving this information from NATA, may decide whether or not to allow the information to be revealed. If the reporting member decides that the necessary information must remain confidential, NATA may be required to close the unfinished investigation for lack of necessary information. NATA members are strongly encouraged to provide information, with as much detail as possible, in writing.

D.   *Investigation*

1. Whenever the Chair of the Investigative Panel receives allegations which in his or her judgment sufficiently and meaningfully raise the possibility of violations of Sections III A (1)-(6), above, by an NATA applicant or member, the Investigative Panel, through a Presiding Panel composed of three (3) members appointed by the Chair, shall conduct a preliminary inquiry into the mat-

ter. Upon commencing such a preliminary inquiry, the Chair of the Investigative Panel shall by certified mail, return receipt requested, notify the NATA applicant or member in question that such an inquiry is being conducted and shall state the provisions of the Membership Standards relating to said preliminary inquiry. This notification shall be provided in or consistent with the form specified by NATA's counsel, and shall be reviewed by NATA's Executive Director or counsel prior to mailing.

2. If the three-member Presiding Investigative Panel by majority vote determines that there is good cause to believe that a more formal and thorough investigation need be conducted, such an investigation shall commence. If such an investigation commences, the Chair of the Presiding Investigative Panel shall by certified mail, return receipt requested, so notify the NATA applicant or member in question and shall specify the pro visions of the Membership Standards relating to said formal investigation.

3. If the three-member Presiding Investigative Panel by majority vote determines that no good cause exists to question compliance with the relevant Membership Standards, no further action shall be taken. The inquiry shall be closed, and the Chair of the Presiding Investigative Panel shall, by certified mail, return receipt requested, so notify the NATA applicant or member in question, the Chair of NATA's Ethics Committee and NATA's Executive Director.

4. If, after formal investigation, the three-member Presiding Investigative Panel by majority vote determines that there is good cause to believe that the NATA applicant or member in question has violated one or more of the Membership Standards, the Chair of the Presiding Investigative Panel shall, after appropriate review by counsel, forward to said NATA applicant or

member by certified mail, return receipt requested, a detailed statement ("Statement of Allegations") setting forth:

(a) The Membership Standards allegedly violated;

(b) A summary of the Presiding Investigative Panel's allegations and charges;

(c) A summary of the evidence establishing the alleged violations of the Membership Standards;

(d) The possible sanctions for the alleged violations;

(e) Notification that the NATA applicant or member in question has the right to legal counsel in all subsequent proceedings;

(f) Notification that the NATA applicant or member in question has the right to request an oral and/or written hearing before the NATA Fact-Finding Panel with respect to the Statement of Allegations, with said applicant or member bearing his or her own expenses for such hearings;

(g) Notification that the NATA applicant or member in question shall have twenty-one (21) days after receipt of the Statement of Allegations:

   i. to notify the Panel if he or she disputes the allegations or possible sanctions set forth in the Statement of Allegations;

   ii. to submit a brief written response setting forth the applicant's or member's reasons for disputing the Statement of Allegations; and

   iii. to request an oral and/or written hearing;

(h) Notification that the NATA applicant or member in question, in any matter in which a possible sanction is one of those listed in Sections III G 2 (a)-(e) below, may appear in person before the Presiding Fact-Finding Panel with the assistance of counsel, may make opening statements, present documents and testimony, examine and cross-examine witnesses under oath, make closing statements, and present written submissions on his or her behalf;

(i)   Notification that the NATA applicant or member in question, in any matter in which the possible sanctions are only those listed in Sections III G 2 (f)-(i) below, may request an oral hearing by telephone conference call with the Presiding Fact-Finding Panel, at which time the NATA applicant or member in question may participate with the assistance of counsel, may make appropriate statements or arguments, and may respond to questions from the Presiding Panel;

(j)   Notification that the NATA applicant or member in question may in any matter, if he or she wishes, waive oral hearing and merely submit written materials to the Presiding Fact-Finding Panel in response to the Statement of Allegations, on a schedule to be established by the Fact-Finding Panel;

(k)   Notification that the establishment of the truth of the Statement of Allegations or the failure to respond thereto may result in the levying of any or all of the sanctions listed in the Statement of Allegations upon the NATA applicant or member in question;

(l)   Notification that if the NATA applicant or member in question does not dispute the Statement of Allegations, he or she consents that the Investigative Panel may refer the matter to the Fact-Finding Panel which may render a decision and levy appropriate sanctions.

5. If the NATA applicant or member in question disputes in any way the allegations or sanctions set forth in the Statement of Allegations, the Chair of the Investigative

Panel shall forward the matter and the entire record thereof to the Chair of the Fact-Finding Panel.

6. All decisions of the three member Investigative Panel shall be considered the decisions of the entire Investigative Panel.

E.   *Fact Finding*

1. After receipt of the record of a matter from the Chair of the Investigative Panel, the Chair of the Fact-Finding Panel shall with reasonable expedition:
    (a) appoint three members of the Panel, two of whom are Ethics Committee members, to preside over the matter;
    (b) schedule an appropriate hearing before the Presiding Panel members;
    (c) forward to the NATA applicant or member in question by certified mail, return receipt requested, a Notice of Hearing setting forth the identity of the Presiding Panel members and the date of the hearing.

2. The Fact-Finding Presiding Panel shall tape record all oral hearings.

3. In any matter in which a hearing is requested and a possible sanction is one of those listed in Sections III G 2 (a)-(e) below, the NATA and the applicant or member in question may make opening statements, present documents and testimony, examine and cross-examine witnesses under oath, make closing statements, and tender written submissions as permitted and scheduled by the Presiding Panel member. In all other matters in which a hearing is requested, both NATA and the applicant or member in question shall submit their contentions in writing as and when directed by the Presiding Panel members.

4. The Presiding Panel members shall determine all matters relating to hearing. All decisions of the Presiding

Panel shall be considered the decisions of the entire Fact-Finding Panel.

5. If the Presiding Panel members, after a full and fair hearing, determine that the preponderance of the evidence does not establish any violation of the Membership Standards, no further action shall be taken. The case shall be closed, and the Presiding Panel shall, by certified mail, return receipt requested, so notify the NATA applicant or member in question, the Chair of NATA's Ethics Committee and NATA's Executive Director.

6. If the Presiding Panel members, after a full and fair hearing, determine that the preponderance of the evidence does establish that a provision of the Membership Standards has been violated, the Chair of the Presiding Panel shall prepare a written decision setting forth:

   (a) Membership Standards that have been violated;

   (b) findings of fact establishing said violations;

   (c) appropriate sanctions; and

   (d) other relevant and appropriate information.

7. The Chair of the Fact-Finding Panel shall promptly forward a copy of the Presiding Panel's decision to the NATA applicant or member in question by certified mail, return receipt requested. The Chair shall also notify the NATA applicant or member in question in writing that he or she has the right to appeal the decision by submitting to the Chair of the Fact-Finding Panel a Notice of Appeal within ten (10) days of his or her receipt of the decision.

8. Upon receipt of a Notice of Appeal in any case, the Chair of the Fact-Finding Panel shall forward said Notice and the rest of the record of the case to the Chair of the Appellate Panel.

9. In every case in which the NATA applicant or member in question chooses not to appeal the decision of the

presiding member of the Fact-Finding Presiding Panel, that decision shall be the final decision in the matter.

10. When a decision of the Presiding Fact-Finding Panel is final, and the NATA applicant or member chooses not to appeal the decision, the Chair of the Fact-Finding Panel shall notify the Chair of the Investigative Panel, the Chair of the Ethics Committee, and NATA's Executive Director that a final decision has been reached, and shall notify each as to the nature of the decision. The Chair of the Fact-Finding Panel shall then turn over the complete file of the case to NATA's Executive Director.

F. *Evidence*

Formal rules of evidence shall not apply in any hearing before Fact-Finding Presiding Panels. Relevant evidence shall be admitted in all hearings. The Presiding Panel member shall resolve all questions disputed at the hearing, and shall notify counsel of its decisions with appropriate opportunity for review, before any sanctions are levied.

G. *Sanctions*

1. Sanctions for violations of any Membership Standard shall in all cases be reasonable in all the circumstances.
2. Such sanctions may include one or more of the following:
    (a) denial of eligibility;
    (b) cancellation of membership;
    (c) non-renewal of membership;
    (d) suspension of membership;
    (e) public censure;
    (f) private reprimand;
    (g) required training or other corrective action;
    (h) written reports with limited circulation; and
    (i) conditions related to the above.

H. *Appeal*

1   Upon receipt of a Notice of Appeal and the remaining record of a case from the Chair of the Fact-Finding Panel, the Chair of the Appellate Panel shall:

(a)   appoint three members of the Appellate Panel (one Ethics Committee member, one at-large member, and one director from the Board) to preside over the appeal;

(b)   set a briefing schedule pursuant to which both NATA and the appealing NATA applicant or member may present their contentions in writing to the Presiding Panel with respect to the decision of the Fact-Finding Panel. For purposes of this presentation, NATA shall be represented by a member of the Ethics Committee, selected by the Committee, who is not or was not sitting on any panel involved with the case being appealed, and the written submission of that representative shall have been reviewed by NATA's Executive Director and approved by NATA's counsel; and

(c)   set a date for oral hearing either in person or by telephone conference call at the option of NATA, taking into account the seriousness of the allegations and the wishes of the NATA applicant or member. At the hearing, both NATA and the appealing NATA applicant or member may participate with counsel before the Presiding Panel.

(d)   Formal rules of evidence shall not apply in any hearing before the Presiding Appellate Panel. Relevant evidence shall be admitted in all hearings. The Presiding Panel members shall resolve all questions disputed at the hearing, and shall notify counsel of its decisions with appropriate opportunity for review, before any sanctions are levied.

2. After oral hearing and due consideration, the Presiding Panel shall render a decision in writing affirming, reversing, or modifying the decision of the Fact-Finding Panel. The decision of the Presiding Panel shall be considered the decision of the entire Appellate Panel. The decision of the Presiding Panel members shall set forth the Panel's factual findings as well as the rationale for decision with respect to any violations of the Membership Standards and the levying of sanctions.

3. In every case in which an NATA applicant or member exercises his or her appellate rights, the decision of the Appellate Panel shall be the final decision in the matter.

IV. Confidentiality of Proceedings

All proceedings before the Investigative, Fact-Finding, and Appellate Panels shall in all respects be confidential, except where:

A. Disclosure is required by law or agreement; or

B. A proceeding results in a final decision levying one or more of the sanctions listed in Sections III G 2 (a) - (e), above. In each such case, the identity of the NATA applicant or member in question, the provisions of the Membership Standards that have been violated, and the sanctions levied may be made public.

V. Reinstatement of Eligibility or Membership

A. If eligibility is denied or membership canceled or not renewed on grounds set forth at II(A)-(C) or III(A)(1) - (6), eligibility or membership may be reconsidered on the following basis:

    1. In the event of a felony conviction directly related to public health or athletic care or education, no

earlier than one (1) year from the exhaustion of appeals, completion of sentence, or completion of parole, whichever is later; or

2. In any other event, no earlier than one (1) year from the final decision of ineligibility, cancellation, or non-renewal.

B. In addition to other facts required by NATA, the NATA applicant or member in question must fully set forth the circumstances of the decision denying eligibility or canceling or not renewing membership, as well as all relevant facts and circumstances since the decision. The applicant must submit one copy of this material to NATA's Executive Director and one copy to the Chair of the Ethics Committee.

C. In such cases the NATA applicant or member in question bears the burden of demonstrating by clear and convincing evidence that the individual has been rehabilitated, does not pose a danger to others, and deserves NATA membership in all the circumstances.

D. If the Ethics Committee concludes that the NATA applicant or member has met his or her burden of demonstrating by clear and convincing evidence that he or she has been rehabilitated, it will advise the NATA applicant or member and NATA's Executive Director of this fact in writing and specify the date on which the NATA applicant or member's reinstatement or membership becomes effective.

E. If the Ethics Committee concludes that this burden has not been met, it will so advise the Executive Director, who will, with legal counsel, review the decision to ensure that it is consistent with NATA's legal obligations and restrictions. If the Executive Director concludes that this decision is consistent with these obligations and restrictions, he or she will submit the decision to the NATA Board of Directors for ratification by majority vote.

F. If the NATA Executive Director and legal counsel conclude that the decision of the Ethics Committee is not consistent with NATA's legal obligations and restrictions, it will so advise the Ethics Committee and instruct the Committee as to its alternatives.

G. The applicant will be advised promptly of any decision described in Sections V (D) and (E) made by the Ethics Committee, Executive Director, or the Board of Directors.

NATIONAL ATHLETIC TRAINERS' ASSOCIATION MEMBER/APPLICANT ETHICS COMMITTEE

Investigative Panel

9 Members, 3 Preside Over Case
Preliminary Investigation:
- No good cause found for formal investigation—CASE CLOSED
- Good cause found for formal investigation, case forwarded to—FACT-FINDING PANEL

Fact-Finding Panel

7 Members, 3 Preside Over Case
Schedule Hearing:
- No violation found—CASE CLOSED
- Violation found—Member has 10 days to appeal
- Appellate Panel
- No Appeal—THIS IS A FINAL DECISION

Appellate Panel

9 Members, 3 Preside Over Case
Schedule Briefing, Session, Oral Arguments
   Decision:
- Affirmed—Sanctions levied
- Modified
- Reversed
- Case Closed—THIS IS A FINAL DECISION

INVESTIGATIVE PANEL

Preliminary Investigation:
- •3 Members Serve on Panel
- • Member notified by mail of inquiry
- •Letter first approved by
  NATA Executive Director
  and Counsel

Good Cause for Formal Investigation
Notify member in writing of:
- •Alleged violations
- • Panel's allegations
- • Evidence
- • Possible sanctions
- • Member's rights to legal counsel
- • Member has 21 days to respond
- • Member may waive oral hearing and submit written materials
- •Failure to respond may result in the levying of any or all sanctions

All materials sent to Fact-Finding Panel

No Good Cause for Formal
Investigation

Case Closed

Member Notified in Writing

FACT-FINDING PANEL

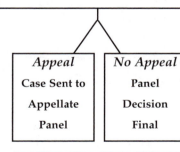

Case Received:
- 3 Member Panel
- Schedule Hearing
- Notify Member

Violation of Standards
Written statement prepared:
- Violations
- Evidence
- Sanctions
- Other Information

Statement mailed to member

Appeal
Case Sent to Appellate Panel

No Appeal
Panel Decision Final

No Violation of Standards

Case Closed

Member Notified in Writing

APPELLATE PANEL

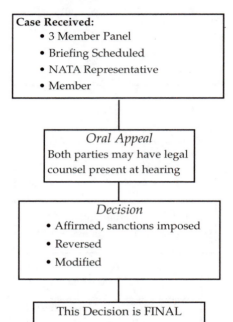

Case Received:
- 3 Member Panel
- Briefing Scheduled
- NATA Representative
- Member

Oral Appeal
Both parties may have legal counsel present at hearing

Decision
- Affirmed, sanctions imposed
- Reversed
- Modified

This Decision is FINAL

Reprinted with permission from:

N A T A

National Athletic
Trainers' Association

2952 Stemmons Freeway • Dallas, Texas 75247
(214) 637-6282

Appendix 20

Weights and Measurements

Reprinted with permission from Bottomley J. *Quick Reference Dictionary for Physical Therapy*. Thorofare, NJ: SLACK Incorporated; 2000.

English System

Linear Measure
12 inches = 1 foot
3 feet = 1 yard (0.9144 meter)
5.5 yards = 1 rod
40 rods = 1 furlong/220 yards
8 furlongs = 1 statute mile/1760 yards
5280 feet = 1 statute or land mile
3 miles = 1 league
6,076.11549 feet = 1 international nautical mile (1852 meters)

Dry Measure
3 teaspoons = 1 tablespoon
12 tablespoons = 1 cup (16 tablespoons liquid = 1 cup)
4 tbsp. = ¼ cup
4 oz. = ½ cup
8 oz. = 1 cup
2 cups = 1 pint
2 pints = 1 quart
4 quarts = 1 gallon
8 quarts = 1 peck
4 pecks = 1 bushel/2150.42 cubic inches
16 oz. = 1 lb.

Angular and Circular Measure
60 seconds = 1 minute
60 minutes = 1 degree
90 degrees = 1 right angle
180 degrees = 1 straight angle
360 degrees = 1 circle

Square Measure
144 square inches = 1 square foot
9 square feet = 1 square yard
30.25 square yards = 1 square rod
160 square rods = 1 acre
640 acres = 1 square mile

Troy Weight
24 grains = 1 pennyweight
20 pennyweights = 1 ounce
12 ounces = 1 pound, Troy

Cubic Measure
1728 cubic inches = 1 cubic foot
27 cubic feet = 1 cubic yard

Liquid Measure
1 teaspoon = 1/8 oz
3 teaspoons = 1 tablespoon
16 tablespoons = 1 cup (12 tablespoons dry = 1 cup)
16 oz. = 1 pint
2 pints = 1 quart
1 quart = .946 liters
4 quarts = 1 gallon/231 cubic inches

Avoirdupois Weight
27.34375 grains = 1 dram
16 drams = 1 ounce
16 ounces = 1 pound/0.45359237 kilogram

100 pounds = 1 short hundredweight
20 short hundredweights = 1 short ton

The Metric System

Linear Measure
10 millimeters = 1 centimeter
10 centimeters = 1 decimeter
10 decimeters = 1 meter
10 meters = 1 dekameter
10 dekameters = 1 hectometer
10 hectometers = 1 kilometer

Liquid Measure
10 milliliters = 1 centiliter
10 centiliters = 1 deciliter
10 deciliters = 1 liter
10 liters = 1 dekaliter
10 dekaliters = 1 hectoliter
10 hectoliters = 1 kiloliter

Square Measure
100 square millimeters = 1 square centimeter
100 square centimeters = 1 square decimeter
100 square decimeters = 1 square meter
100 square meters = 1 square dekameter
100 square dekameters = 1 square hectometer
100 square hectometers = 1 square kilometer

Weights
10 milligrams = 1 centigram
10 centigrams = 1 decigram
10 decigrams = 1 gram
10 grams = 1 dekagram
10 dekagrams = 1 hectogram

10 hectograms = 1 kilogram
100 kilograms = 1 quintal
10 quintals = 1 ton

Cubic Measure
1000 cubic millimeters = 1 cubic centimeter
1000 cubic centimeters = 1 cubic decimeter
1000 cubic decimeters = 1 cubic meter

English and Metric Conversion

Linear Measure
1 centimeter = 0.3937 inch
1 inch = 2.54 centimeters
1 foot = 0.3048 meter
1 meter = 39.37 inches/1.0936 yards
1 yard = 0.9144 meter
1 kilometer = 0.621 mile
1 mile = 1.609 kilometers

Square Measure
1 square centimeter = 0.1550 square inch
1 square inch = 6.452 square centimeters
1 square foot = 0.0929 square meter
1 square meter = 1.196 square yards
1 square yard = 0.8361 square meter
1 hectare = 2.47 acres
1 acre = 0.4047 hectare
1 square kilometer = 0.386 square mile
1 square mile = 2.59 square kilometers

Weight Measure
1 gram = 0.03527 ounce
1 ounce = 28.35 grams
1 kilogram = 2.2046 pounds
1 pound = 0.4536 kilogram

1 metric ton = 0.98421 English ton
1 English ton = 1.016 metric tons

Volume Measure
1 cubic centimeter = 0.061 cubic inch
1 cubic inch = 16.39 cubic centimeters
1 cubic foot = 0.0283 cubic meter
1 cubic meter = 1.308 cubic yards
1 cubic yard = 0.7646 cubic meter
1 liter = 1.0567 quarts
1 quart dry = 1.101 liters
1 quart liquid = 0.9463 liter
1 gallon = 3.78541 liters
1 peck = 8.810 liters
1 hecroliter = 2.8375 bushels

BIBLIOGRAPHY

American Academy of Orthopedic Surgeons. *Joint Motion: Method of Measuring and Recording.* Chicago, Ill: AAOS; 1965.

American Medical Association. *Guide to the Evaluation of Permanent Impairment.* 3rd ed. Chicago, Ill: AMA; 1988.

Bantam Medical Dictionary. New York, NY: Bantam Books Inc; 1982.

Bottomley JM. *Quick Reference Dictionary for Physical Therapy.* Thorofare, NJ: SLACK Incorporated; 2000.

Cantu RC. Posttraumatic retrodgrade and anterograde amnesia: pathophysiology and implications in grading and safe return to play. *Journal of Athletic Training.* 2001; 36:3.

Cantu RC. Return to play guidelines after head injury. *Clin Sports Med.* 1998;17:45-60.

Clemente CD. *Anatomy: A Regional Atlas of the Human Body.* Baltimore, Md: Urban & Schwarzenberg; 1987.

Colorado Medical Society and Sports Medicine Committee. Guidelines for the management of concussion in sports. *Colo Med.* 1990;87:4.

Guskiewicz KM, Perrin DH. Research and clinical applications of assessing balance. *Journal of Sport Rehabilitation.* 1996;5:45-63.

Harmon KG. Assessment and management of concussion in sports. *Am Fam Physician.* 1999;60:887-894.

Hollinshead WH, Rosse C. *Textbook of Anatomy.* 4th ed. Philadelphia, Pa: Harper Row Publ.; 1985.

Houglum PA. *Therapeutic Exercise for Athletic Injuries.* Champaign, Ill: Human Kinetics; 2001.

Jacobs K, Jacobs L. *Quick Reference Dictionary for Occupational Therapy.* 3rd ed. Thorofare, NJ: SLACK Incorporated; 2001.

Jenkins DB. *Hollinshead's Functional Anatomy of the Limbs and Back.* 7th ed. Philadelphia, Pa: WB Saunders Co; 1998.

Kapanji IA. *Physiology of the Joints Volumes 1 and 2.* 2nd ed. London, England: Churchill Livingstone; 1982.

Kendall FP, McCreary EK, Provance PG. *Muscles: Testing and Function.* Baltimore, Md: Williams and Wilkins; 1993.

Kettenbach G. *Writing SOAP Notes.* 2nd ed. Philadelphia, Pa: FA Davis Co; 1990.

King MA. Core stability: creating a foundation for functional rehabilitation. *Athletic Therapy Today.* 2000; 5(2):6-13.

King MA. Functional stability for the upper quarter. *Athletic Therapy Today.* 2000; 5(2):17-21.

Knight KL. Guidelines for rehabilitation of sports injuries. *Clin Sports Med.* 1985;4:405-416.

Kreighbaum E, Barthels KM. *Biomechanics: A Qualitative Approach for Studying Human Movement.* 3rd ed. New York, NY: Macmillan; 1990.

LeVeau BF. *Biomechanics of Human Motion.* Philadelphia, Pa: WB Saunders; 1992.

Magee DJ. *Orthopedic Physical Assessment.* 3rd ed. Philadelphia, Pa: WB Saunders; 1997.

McCrea M, Kelly JT, Randolph C. *The Standardized Assessment of Concussion (SAC): Manual for Administration, Scoring, and Interpretation.* Washington, DC: Brain Injury Association; 1997.

McGinnis PM. *Biomechanics of Sport and Exercise.* Champaign, Ill: Human Kinetics; 1999.

McQuade KJ, Smidt GL. Dynamic scapulohumeral rhythm: the effects of external resistance during elevation of the arm in the scapular plane. *J Orthop Sports Phys Ther.* 1998;27(2):125-133.

Prentice WE. *Therapeutic Modalities in Sports Medicine.* 4th ed. Boston, Mass: McGraw Hill Companies Inc; 1999.

Prentice WE. *Therapeutic for Physical Therapists.* 2nd ed. Boston, Mass: McGraw Hill Companies Inc; 2002.

Prentice WE, Arnheim DD. *Principles of Athletic Training.* 10th ed. Boston, Mass: McGraw Hill Companies Inc; 2000.

Random House Webster's Dictionary. 2nd ed. New York, NY: Random House Incorporated; 1996.

Ray R. *Management Strategies in Athletic Training.* 2nd ed. Champaign, Ill: Human Kinetics; 2000.

Riemann BL, Guskiewicz KM. Relationship between clinical and forceplate measures of postural stability. *Journal of Sport Rehabilitation.* 1999; 8(2):1-7.

Schultz SJ, Houglum PA, Perrin DH. *Assessment of Athletic Injuries.* Champaign, Ill: Human Kinetics; 2001.

Starkey C. *Therapeutic Modalities for Athletic Trainers.* Philadelphia, Pa: FA Davis; 1993.

Starkey C, Ryan J. *Evaluation of Orthopedic and Athletic Injuries.* Philadelphia, Pa: FA Davis; 1996.

Stedman's Concise Medical Dictionary for the Health Professions. 3rd ed. Baltimore, Md: Williams & Wilkins; 1997.

Taber's Cyclopedic Medical Dictionary. 19th ed. Philadelphia, Pa: FA Davis; 2001.

Vincent WJ. *Statistics in Kinesiology.* Champaign, Ill: Human Kinetics; 1995.